Color Atlas of Aesthetic Surgery of the Abdomen

H. DANIEL ATWOOD M.D.
6/15/91

Note p. 62 – naval revision, good point made

Color Atlas of Aesthetic Surgery of the Abdomen

Jorge M. Psillakis, M.D.
Erdulfo Appiani, M.D.
Rafael de la Plaza, M.D.

with a Foreword by Robert M. Goldwyn, M.D.

1991
Thieme Medical Publishers, Inc., NEW YORK
Georg Thieme Verlag STUTTGART · NEW YORK

Thieme Medical Publishers, Inc.
381 Park Avenue South
New York, New York 10016

Color Atlas of Aesthetic Surgery of the Abdomen
Jorge M. Psillakis
Erdulfo Appiani
Rafael de la Plaza

Library of Congress Cataloging-in-Publication Data
Psillakis, Jorge M.
Color atlas of aesthetic surgery of the abdomen / Jorge M. Psillakis, Erdulfo Appiani, Rafael de la Plaza: with a foreword by Robert M. Goldwyn.
p. cm.
Includes bibliographical references.
Includes index.
ISBN 0-86577-343-2. —ISBN 3-13-757501-X
1. Abdomen—Surgery—Atlases. 2. Surgery, Plastic—Atlases. I. Appiani, Erdulfo. II. Plaza, Rafael de la. III. Title.
[DNLM: 1. Abdomen—surgery—atlases. 2. Surgery, Plastic—methods—atlases. WI 17 P974c]
RD119.5.A24P75 1991
617.5′50592—dc20
DNLM/DLC
for Library of Congress 90-11265
CIP

Important note: Medicine is an ever-changing science. Research and clinical experience are continually broadening our knowledge, in particular our knowledge of proper treatment and drug therapy. Insofar as this book mentions any dosage or application, readers may rest assured that the authors, editors, and publishers have made every effort to ensure that such references are strictly in accordance with the state of knowledge at the time of production of the book. Nevertheless, every user is requested to carefully examine the manufacturers' leaflets accompanying each drug to check on his own responsibility whether the dosage schedules recommended therein or the contraindications stated by the manufacturers differ from the statements made in the present book. Such examination is particularly important with drugs that are either rarely used or have been newly released on the market.

Printed in the United States of America

5 4 3 2 1

TMP ISBN 0-86577-343-2
GTV ISBN 3-13-757501-X

To the memory of Isabel,
to Eliana,
to Elvira,
and to our patients

Contents

Foreword

Since 1899, when Howard A. Kelly, the eminent gynecologist-obstetrician at Johns Hopkins, performed an abdominal wall "lipectomy," the procedure has changed significantly with respect to both technique and purpose. Originally done as a panniculectomy to relieve dysfunction, this operation became what we plastic surgeons call "abdominoplasty," which unfortunately is known to the public as a "tummy tuck," a label that falsely minimizes its surgical nature and its possible complications. Patients now may seek abdominoplasty not to eliminate deformity but to enhance appearance, which already may be acceptable though perhaps not optimal. It is interesting, however, that Kelly concluded that "quite apart . . . from the tremendous physical and, in some cases, psychical benefit, I personally recommend and would do the operation in extreme cases for the cosmetic effect."

This excellent atlas by Dr. Jorge Psillakis and his colleagues carefully and clearly instructs the reader in the various kinds of abdominoplasty, describing the indications as well as the mechanics, the basic steps as well as the refinements. To any surgeon performing aesthetic surgery of the abdomen, it should be apparent that no single operation can give every patient the best outcome. Too frequently in the past, surgeons imposed their favorite abdominoplasty technique on patients whose anatomic problem necessitated a different approach.

From this well-illustrated book, the reader will receive the distillate of the authors' extensive experience. A critical feature is the detailed description of not just what to do in the operating room but what to look for as one examines the patient preoperatively. In plastic surgery, as in everything else, one must know what is wrong before attempting to correct it. Toward that goal, this admirable volume will prove an indispensable guide.

Robert M. Goldwyn, M.D.
Clinical Professor of Surgery,
Harvard Medical School;
Head, Division of Plastic Surgery,
Beth Israel Hospital

Preface

The goal of this atlas is to put together the knowledge acquired through experience by this century's plastic surgeons in the field of aesthetic surgery of the abdomen, with the intent of writing a "how to do it" atlas rather than an encyclopedic book.

Historically, the evolution of abdominoplasty can be divided into four periods: (1) up to 1962, the goal of such surgery was the reduction of the skin and fat to alleviate the patient's weight excess and to correct musculoaponeurotic flaccidity by plication of the aponeurosis at the "linea alba"; (2) from 1962 to 1974, the objective was aesthetic abdominoplasty with a horizontal suprapubic scar to be hidden by the bikini, associated with the correction of the diastasis of the rectus muscles. In spite of the great advancement of this period, the aesthetic results were unnatural, without details and with a flat appearance, long scars, and elevation of the pubis; (3) in 1974, resection of the oblique muscles was introduced in an effort to obtain a better sculpturing of the abdomen; and (4) after 1980 the defatting of the subcutaneous tissue with knife and liposuction were introduced to rebuild the depressions and elevations in order to enhance the light reflections and shadows for a more pleasant aesthetic result and a smaller scar.

The ideal goal of abdominoplasty today is to reproduce a young and natural appearance. With the various techniques we have to choose from, it is important to be selective in their application in order to obtain a result in which the abdomen will look natural without the stigma of a "plastic surgical abdomen."

To attain this result, we need to keep in mind what we consider to be a beautiful abdomen; we also need to know the artistic anatomy and the role that each layer of the abdominal wall exerts in aesthetic appearance.

In this atlas, we have attempted to present practical ways of performing an abdominoplasty, emphasizing the refinements that will attain beauty rather than the reduction of volume alone.

To facilitate comprehension, the book is divided into sections: in the first chapter, concepts of beauty, light reflections and shadows, and the role that the various anatomic layers exert in the aesthetic appearance are covered; in the second chapter, a detailed preoperative examination of each patient and classification of the deformities we routinely encounter in the office are outlined; in the third chapter, the operative techniques are described; and in the fourth chapter, postoperative care, results, and complications—and how to avoid such complications—are explained.

A bibliography is provided to lead the reader to works of basic importance. We apologize to our friends whose writings have not been included.

We gratefully acknowledge the help of those who made this publication posssible: Dr. Antonio Roberto Bozola for his cooperation in this book; Franz W. Guzmán and Sergio Sanni for their expert drawings; Eliana P. de Almeida for the photographs; Maysa Graham for fine-tuning our English; Rosana Ramos de Almeida for helping to assemble this project in its final stages; and Hilary Evans, Editor in Chief, Thieme Medical Publishers, Inc., and John de Carville, President, de Carville Associates, Inc., for their help and support.

Additional thanks to all our patients for their patience with us and to all of the assistants and residents we have worked with for their interest and help in the care of the patients.

Jorge M. Psillakis, M.D.
Erdulfo Appiani, M.D.
Rafael de la Plaza, M.D.

1

Introduction

CONCEPT OF BEAUTY

The concept of beauty changes with time and geographic regions. This also occurs in relation to the abdomen.

The bone structure of man of the Upper Paleolithic Age, who lived 40,000 years ago, was the same as today, but the morphology of the soft parts of the female body had very exuberant secondary sexual characteristics: abundant adipose tissue on the buttocks, breasts, and abdomen and no waistline. This is demonstrated by the statutes of Venus of Willendorf, Savignano, and Laussel, among others.

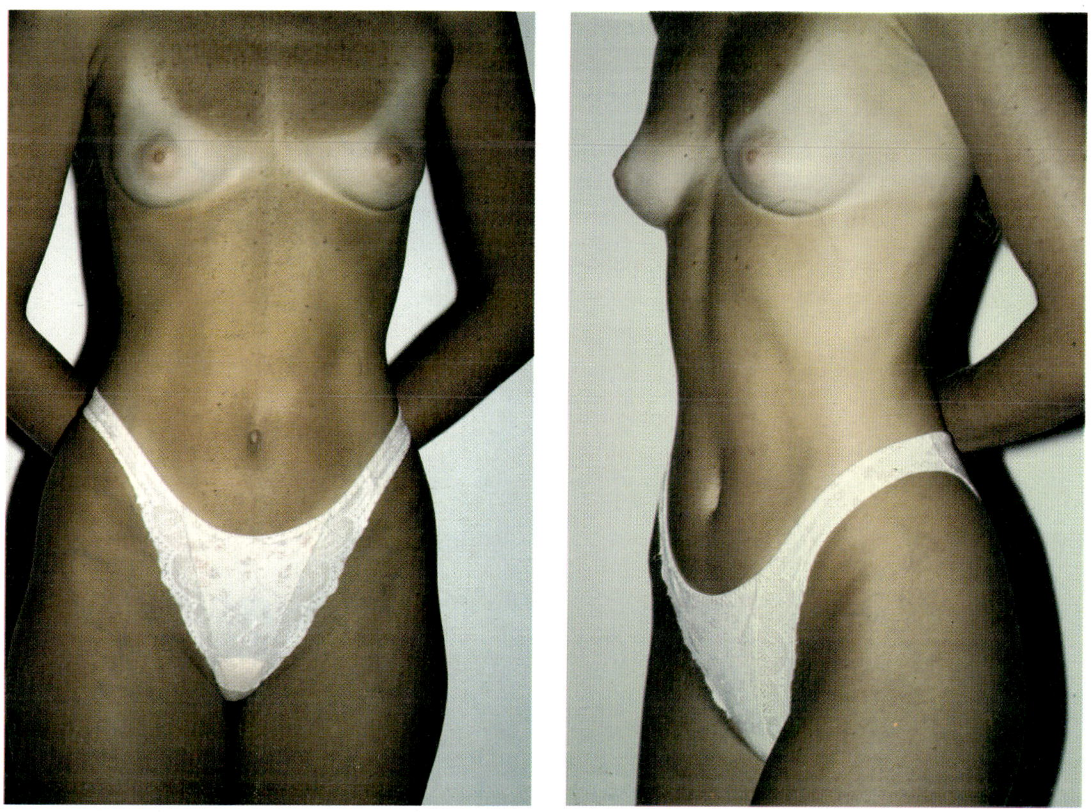

A B

Figure 1–1. A–I: Modern abdomens accepted as the standard of beauty. They are different, but they have in common: medial sulcus in the upper abdomen, two shadows of the semilunar line that join over the pubis, two protuberances between the shadows beginning in the thorax that join under the umbilicus, with a "lyre" shape. Observe that under the umbilicus the abdomen is not flat, but prominent. (*Figure continues*)

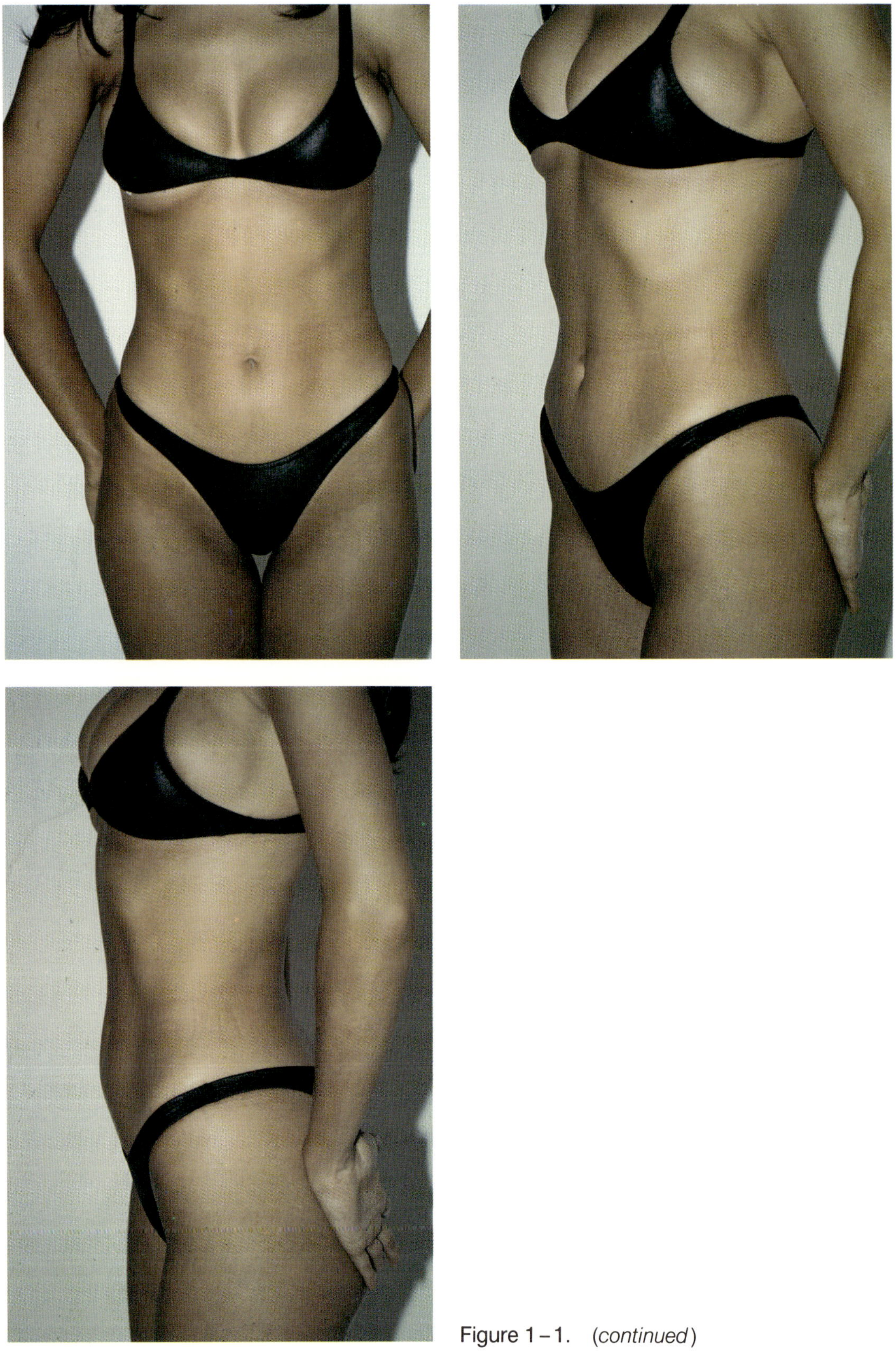

C D E

Figure 1–1. *(continued)*

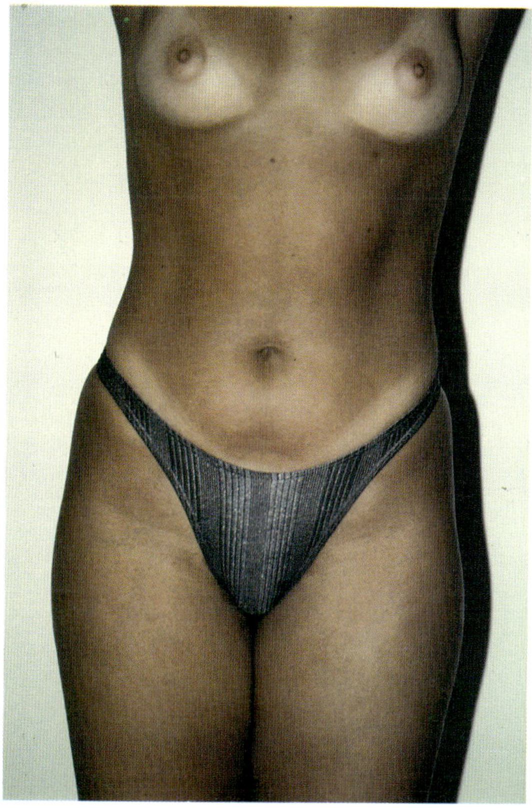
F

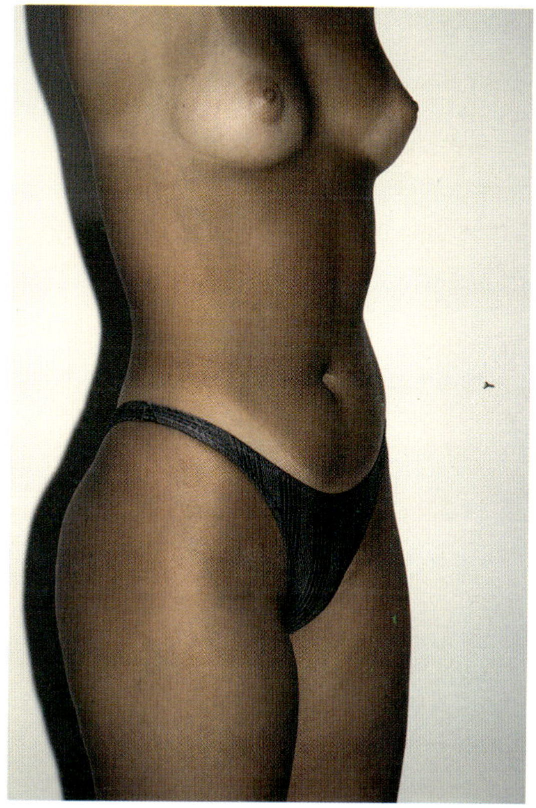
G

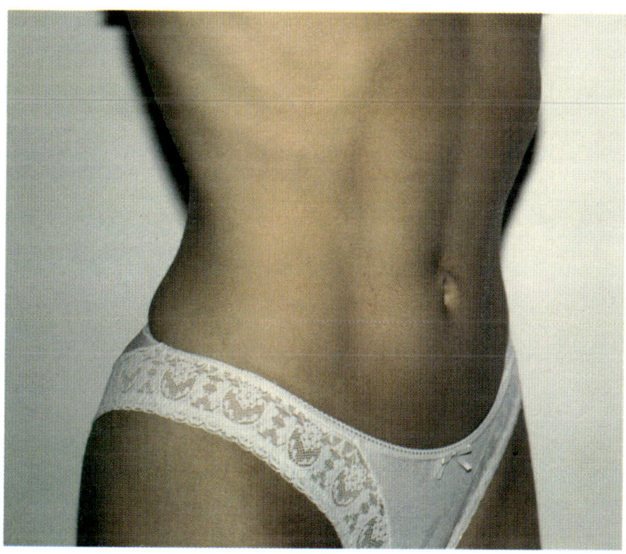
H

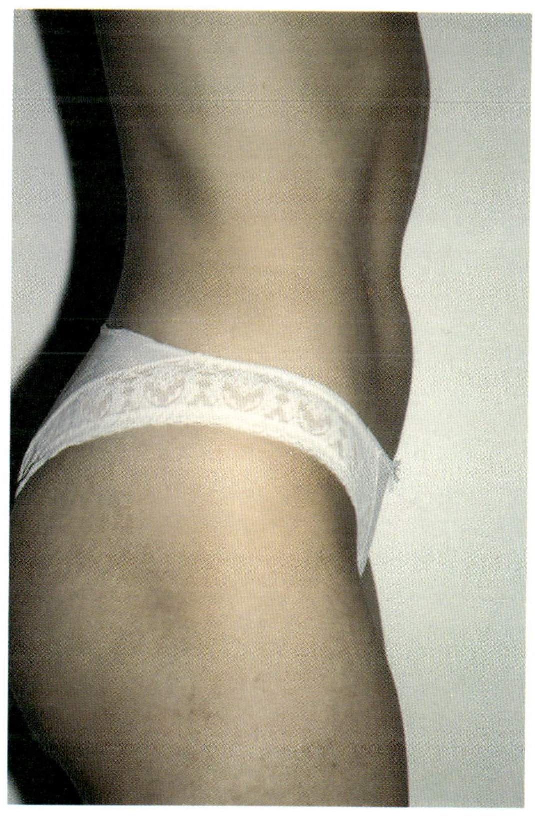
I

Figure 1–1. *(continued)*

During the Greek and Roman periods, female beauty was characterized by a certain amount of adipose tissue uniformly distributed throughout the body, hiding the muscular shape that can be seen in the Aphrodite and Venus statues.

Even in the occidental world, from the Renaissance to the 20th century, female beauty was expressed through more rounded abdomens, thighs, hips, and buttocks, as can be seen in the paintings of Rubens, Rembrandt, and Renoir.

At the present time, the physical form of female beauty is characterized by a graceful silhouette with no adipose tissue, a flat abdomen, and a delicate waist (Fig. 1–1A–I). This aesthetic concept places emphasis on youth and fitness with a "healthy" appearance, in which a flat belly without fat is the goal. The "puffiness" under the umbilicus, always considered a sign of beauty and femininity, has become undesirable. Fat deposits are considered "unhealthy," "nonaesthetic," and "ugly." There is a tendency toward a muscular-type body. We can foresee that the concept of beauty will be that of a more unisex appearance. Progressively, fitness is manifested by seeking to show only the body's muscular structure. Many of us may not agree with this type of contour, but this concept will probably be the ideal goal for a certain period of time.

OBJECTIVE OF ABDOMINOPLASTY

Abdominoplasty previously was a technique whose objective was just to reduce excess skin and fat and the plication of the rectus muscles. This may result in unnatural contours, with a flat abdomen, elevation of the pubis, and a long scar. However, the objective of abdominoplasty today is to treat the various anatomic layers of tissue in order to rebuild the natural prominences so that they will reflect the light and to reshape the depressions so that they will produce shadows.

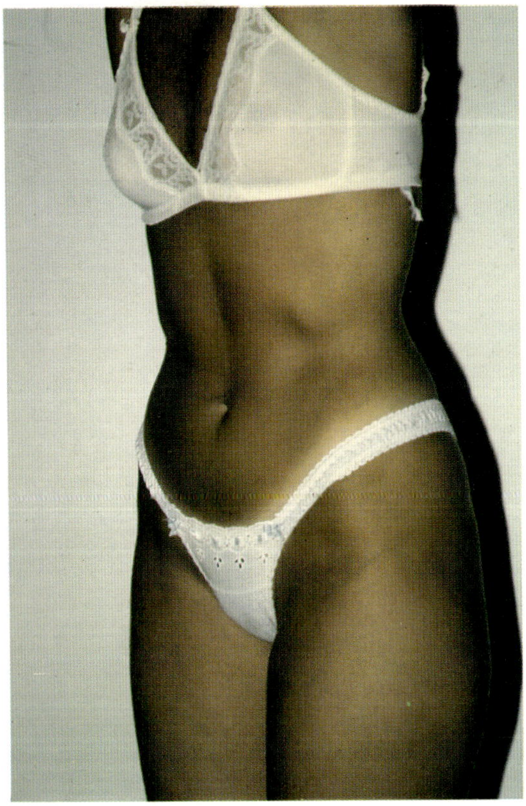

Figure 1–2. In the superior abdomen the detail of the shadow forming the medial sulcus from the xiphoid to the navel is apparent. Also observe the lateral prominences that contrast with the sulcus.

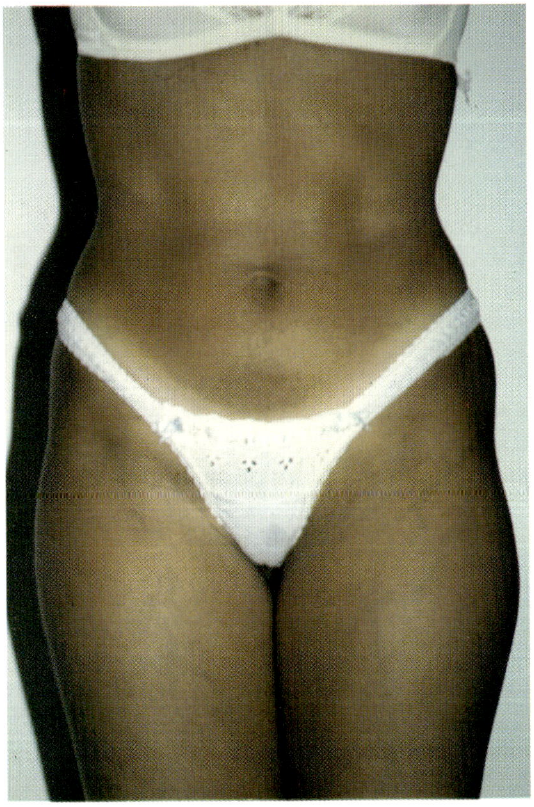

Figure 1–3. Lateral to the medial sulcus, light reflections are produced by the prominences of the rectus muscles. These prominences continue under the umbilicus due to the fat deposits, also producing an area of light reflection.

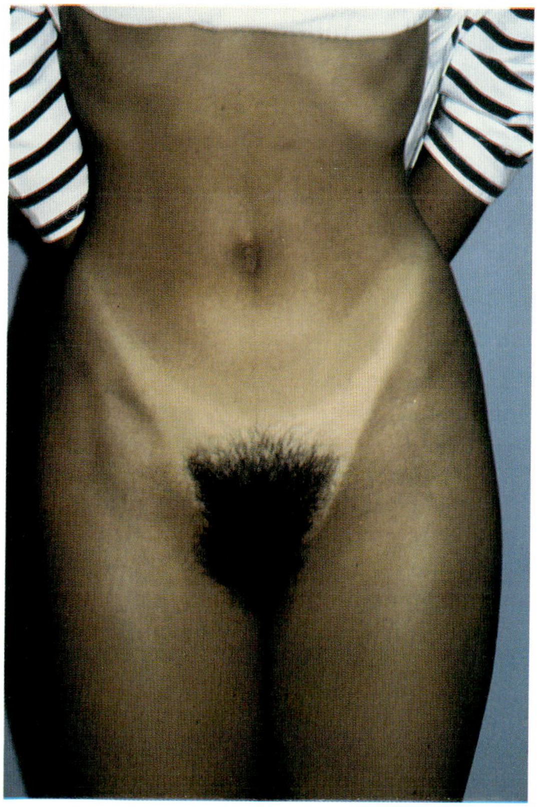

A

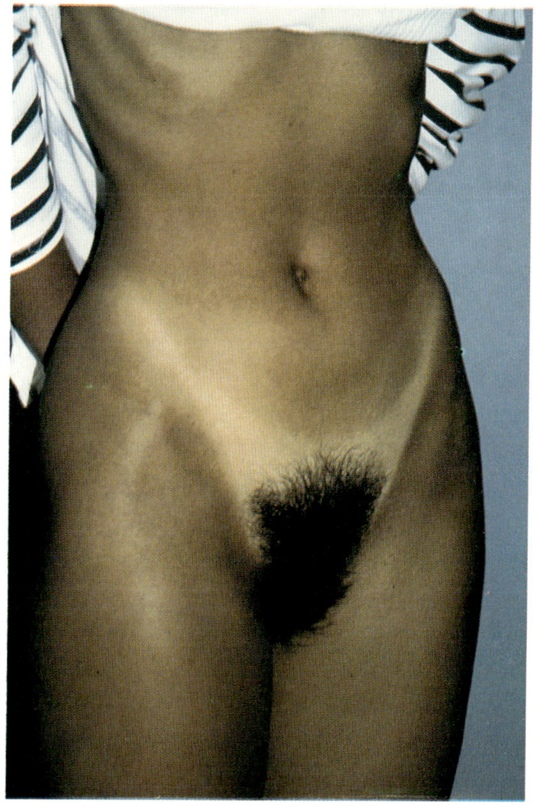

B

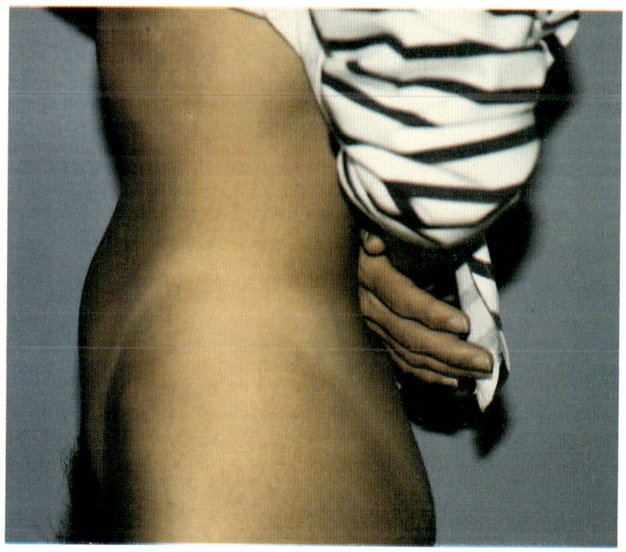

C

Figure 1–4. **A–C:** Two wide strips of shadows in the upper abdomen produced by fixation of the skin at the fascia of the oblique muscle, which is inserted into the external margin of the rectus muscles. Inferiorly it is inserted into the inguinal ligaments and pubis.

THE AESTHETIC ABDOMEN: LIGHT REFLECTIONS AND SHADOWS

The abdominal wall is formed by the relationship between the osteomuscular system, the subcutaneous fibroadipose tissue, and the skin. This relationship gives the appearance of an aesthetic contour with light reflection produced by prominences and shadows resulting from depressions. In the midline from the xiphoid to the navel a shadow is formed by the depression of the medial sulcus (Fig. 1–2). Lateral to this sulcus, there are two vertical wide strip reflections produced by the prominence of the rectus muscle that join under the umbilicus, forming a mound (Fig. 1–3).

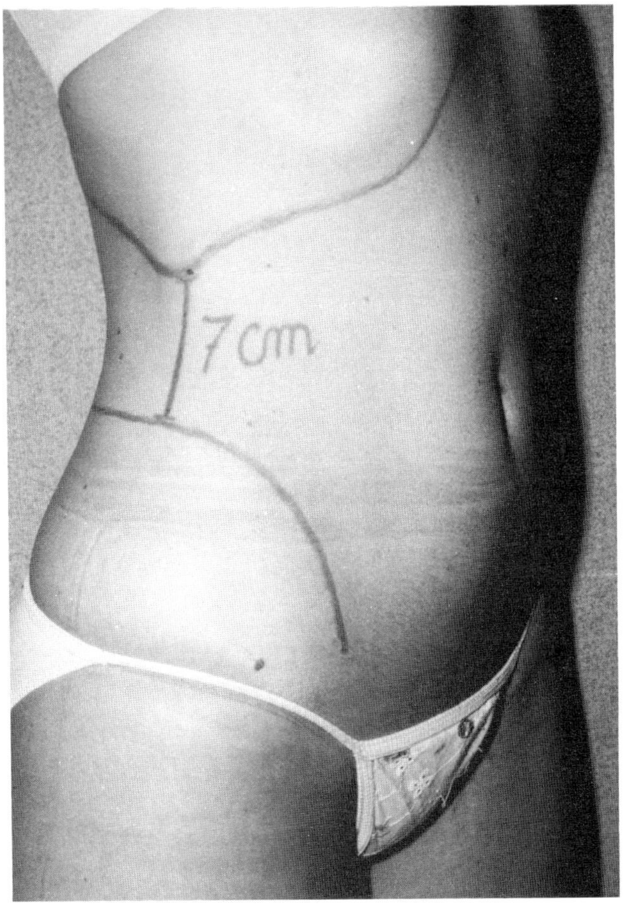

Figure 1–5. The height of the waist measures 7 to 10 cm and is limited by the bony skeleton.

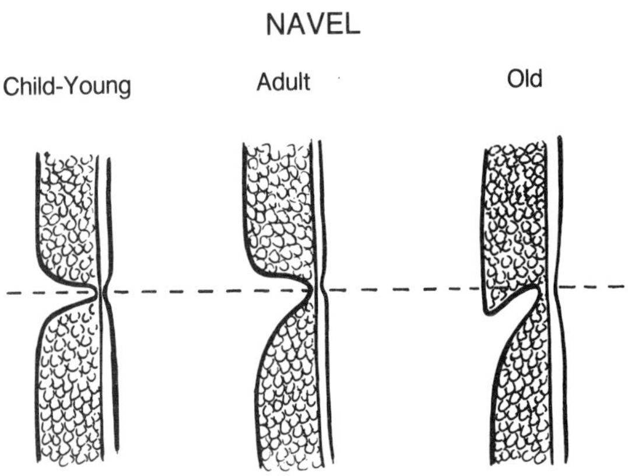

A

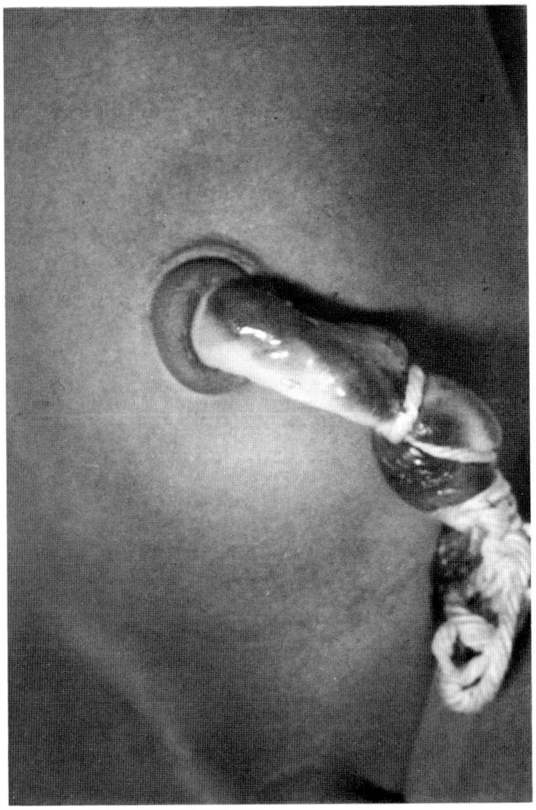

B

Figure 1–6. The umbilicus at various ages. B: 1 week old; C: 1 year old; D: 15 years old; E: 30 years old; and F: 60 years old. (*Figure continues*)

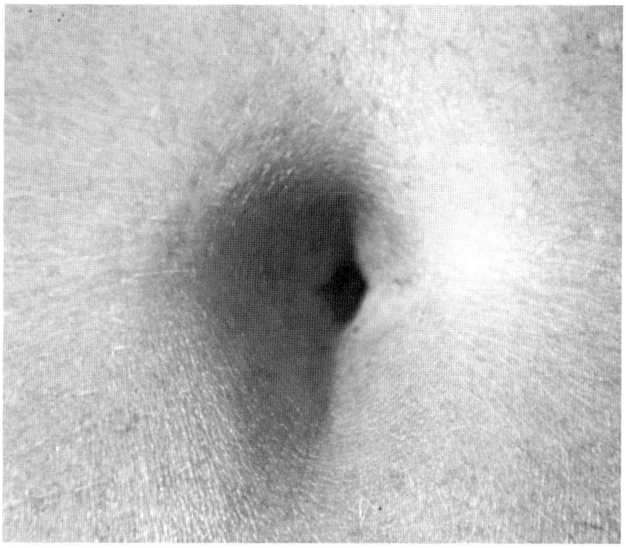
C

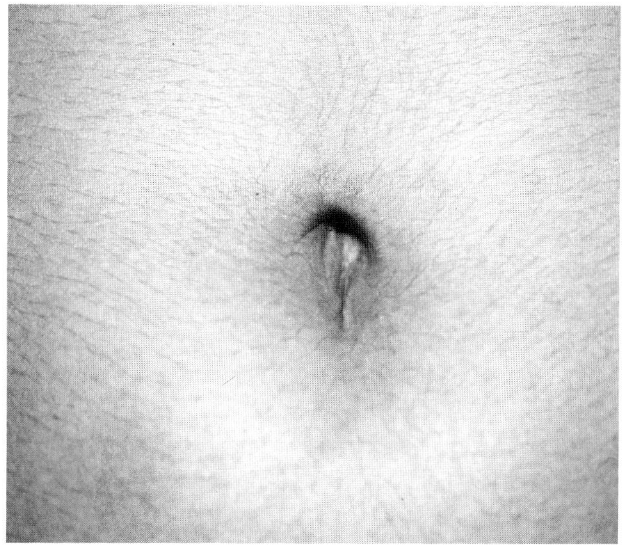
D

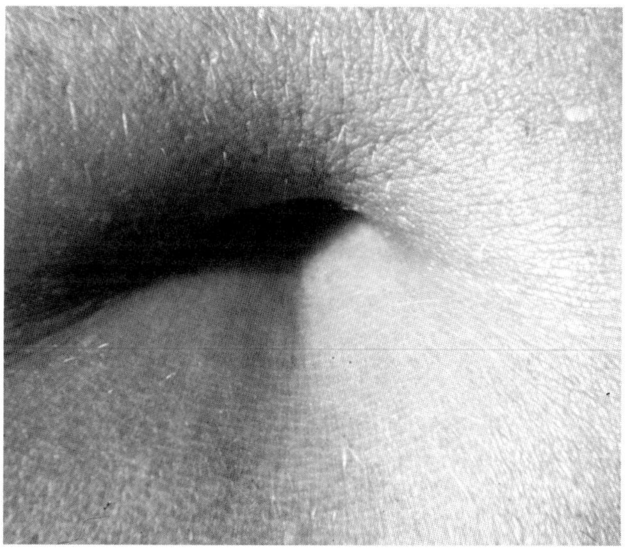
E

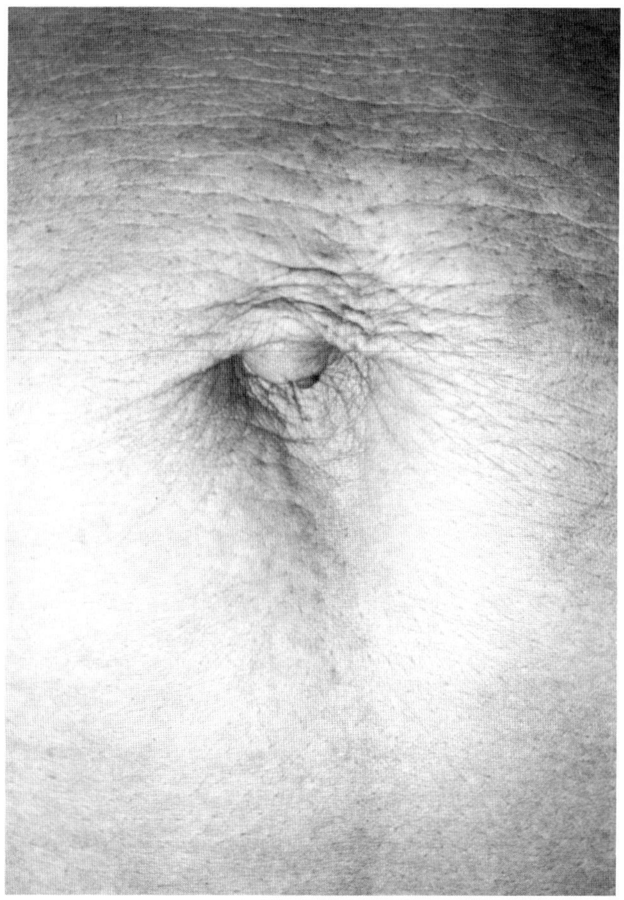
F

Figure 1-6. *(continued)*

More lateral and slightly more posterior to these prominences, there are two wide strips of shadows called "semilunar" sulcus, in "lyre" form, produced by the depressions formed by the insertion of the skin at the fascia of the oblique muscles, which are inserted into the external margin of the rectus muscles and into the inguinal ligaments and pubis (Fig. 1–4A–C). More laterally, the profile of the abdomen is formed by the thoracic cage superiorly, the pelvis inferiorly, and the waist in the middle. The waist extends 7 to 10 cm between the inferior costal ribs and the iliac crest (Fig. 1–5). The shape of the waist is also dependent on the superior aperture of the pelvis. The larger the pelvis, the more accentuated the waist. The waist can be absent when the pelvis is small, when the distance between the pelvis and the ribs is reduced, or when muscular atony or fat deposits are present.

In the inferior extremity of the shadow of the medial sulcus a more accentuated shadow is formed by the triangular depression of the navel. Spatially, it is situated 1 or 2 cm over a transverse plane that corresponds to the third or fourth lumbar vertebra. The shape of the navel varies from person to person and also varies at different ages (Fig. 1–6A–C).

Modifications of the spatial position and thickness of the tissues will alter the aesthetic appearance of the abdomen due to the changes of the light reflections and shadows. Therefore, the basic surgical principle today in abdominoplasty is to sculpture the tissues, reshaping the light reflections and shadows by giving a new tension in the musculoaponeurotic layer, by sculpturing the overlaying fat on the cutaneous envelope, and by resecting excess skin when it is present.

2

Preoperative Evaluation

PATIENT EVALUATION

At the first consultation it is important to listen very carefully and with the utmost attention to the complaints of the patient. In the majority of cases the first complaint is that there is excess fat and skin in the area of the umbilicus. The second complaint is that there is laxity of the skin in the overall abdomen and stria, as well as the flaccidity of the musculoaponeurotic layer. Sometimes the complaint is the excess skin in the upper part of the abdomen over the umbilicus or a bulging epigastric region, not only due to the muscles, but due to the projection of the inferior thoracic cage. Many patients complain that the abdomen is nonaesthetic, with an overall bulging and with excess fat. Less frequently, there are complaints that the waist is too large or has increased after pregnancy. Another frequent complaint is that of scars from previous surgeries: in the infraumbilical area the vertical scar will produce a depression in the midline; in the area of the upper abdomen, it will prevent the patient from wearing a bikini. Sometimes there are hernias due to previous surgeries.

Even though patients are aware of the ideal shape of a beautiful abdomen, they never complain of the loss of the natural "lyre" form due to muscle flaccidity and fat deposits. They will not complain about the disappearance of the superior medial sulcus or the semilunar line, but they know "something" is wrong. We need to keep this in mind during the examination and discuss it with the patient.

The clinical examination must begin with the patient standing nude, exposing the area from immediately under the brassiere to the knees, while wearing only a small bikini covering the pubic area. It is possible to find disposable paper bikinis in the marketplace.

We feel it is better to begin the examination from the back, because the patient is more comfortable at first if they are not looking directly at us. In the dorsal region we note any deviations in the vertebral column, the depth of the lordosis in the lumbar region, and the extent of the projection of the buttocks. The more concave the lumbar region, the more prominent the abdomen will be. These patients will have a prominent abdomen due to the skeletal bone structure, which will limit our final result, since they will always have some anterior prominence.

At this time, we also examine any excess tissue over the hips noting how far back the fullness extends to determine the area that will require liposuction.

From the frontal view, the patient must be examined from the superior to the inferior area, studying first the thoracic cage, the aperture of the angle of the ribs, and the anterior projection of the inferior ribs. This will give an idea of how much we can reduce the projection of the upper abdomen during surgery. The epigastric region is examined in the midline, and we need to determine the amount of excess skin at the central area between the xiphoid and the umbilicus. At this time, we also look for the presence or absence of the medial sulcus. More laterally, we examine the thickness of fat tissue deposit over the rectus muscles and the presence or absence of the semilunar sulcus.

As we move downward, the size of the waist, the excess fat, and the flaccidity of the muscles are noted. At the level of the umbilicus, we examine the shape of the umbilicus, the excess skin immediately over it, as well as the amount of fat surrounding it. To evaluate the amount of cutaneous tissue to be resected, the infraumbilical skin is pinched with the fingers of both hands in a horizontal direction (Fig. 2–1). This maneuver gives us an idea of the width and length of the skin to be resected. The same maneuver is performed in the upper abdomen. If there is a great excess in this area, the resection of the skin in the lower abdomen must be done from the pubis to the navel, or we may perform a reverse abdominoplasty. The pubis is also examined to see the amount of fat that may need reduction for a better final result. The patient is then flexed to allow the examination of the flaccidity of the skin, its mobility in relation to the musculoaponeurotic plane, as well as the possibility of eventrations.

From a profile view, we examine the design of the abdominal arch and its relation to the lumbodorsal region. The more accentuated the convexity of the abdominal arch, and the more flacid the rectus muscles, probably the greater the diastasis between them. The patient is then flexed to allow us to examine the tension of the musculoaponeurotic layer.

To detect the tension of the muscles, we perform two maneuvers: while standing up, the patient is asked to retract the abdomen, and while lying down, the patient is asked to elevate both legs at the same time.

After specific examinations of all areas, a general overview of the abdomen is made, examining again the semilunar line, the fat deposits in specific areas, and the lateral contouring of the waist and hips. This general overview added to our previous specific examinations will allow a classification of the abdomen in each case.

Standard photographs of the patient must be taken in frontal and at 90° and 45° angles. The photograph needs to show the area from the upper part of the thigh to the breast. The arms must be flexed posteriorly with the hands at the level of the buttocks.

CLASSIFICATION OF ABDOMINAL AESTHETIC DEFORMITIES AND SUMMARY OF SURGICAL TREATMENT

Type I

This first category consists of young nulliparous women with normal skin and muscle tone, but with an excess of fat in the subcutaneous tissue more evident in the infraumbilical area (Figs. 2–2 to 2–4). These patients are treated by suction-as-

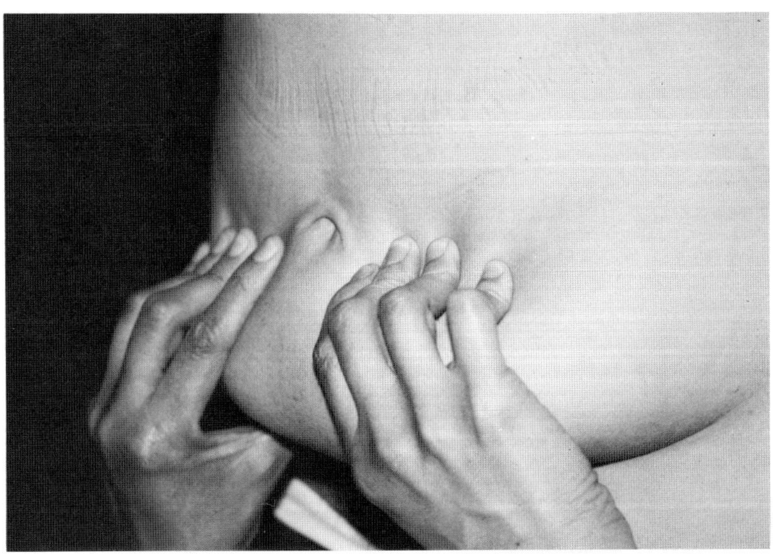

Figure 2–1. The excess of cutaneous tissue under the umbilicus is determined by pinching the lower abdomen.

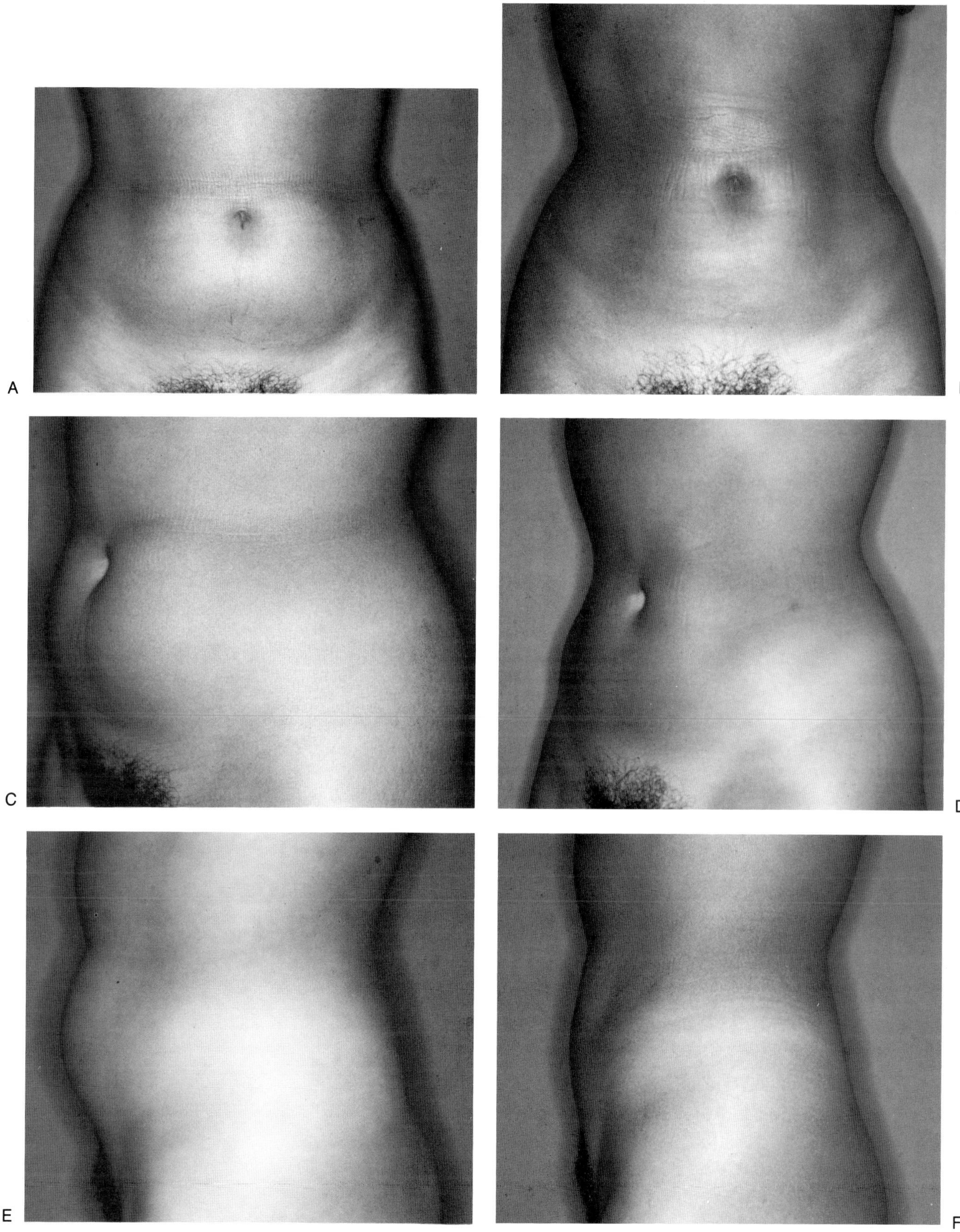

Figure 2–2. **A, C, E:** Type I: with peri- and infraumbilical fat; treated only with suction-assisted lipectomy. **B, D, F:** Six-month postoperative result.

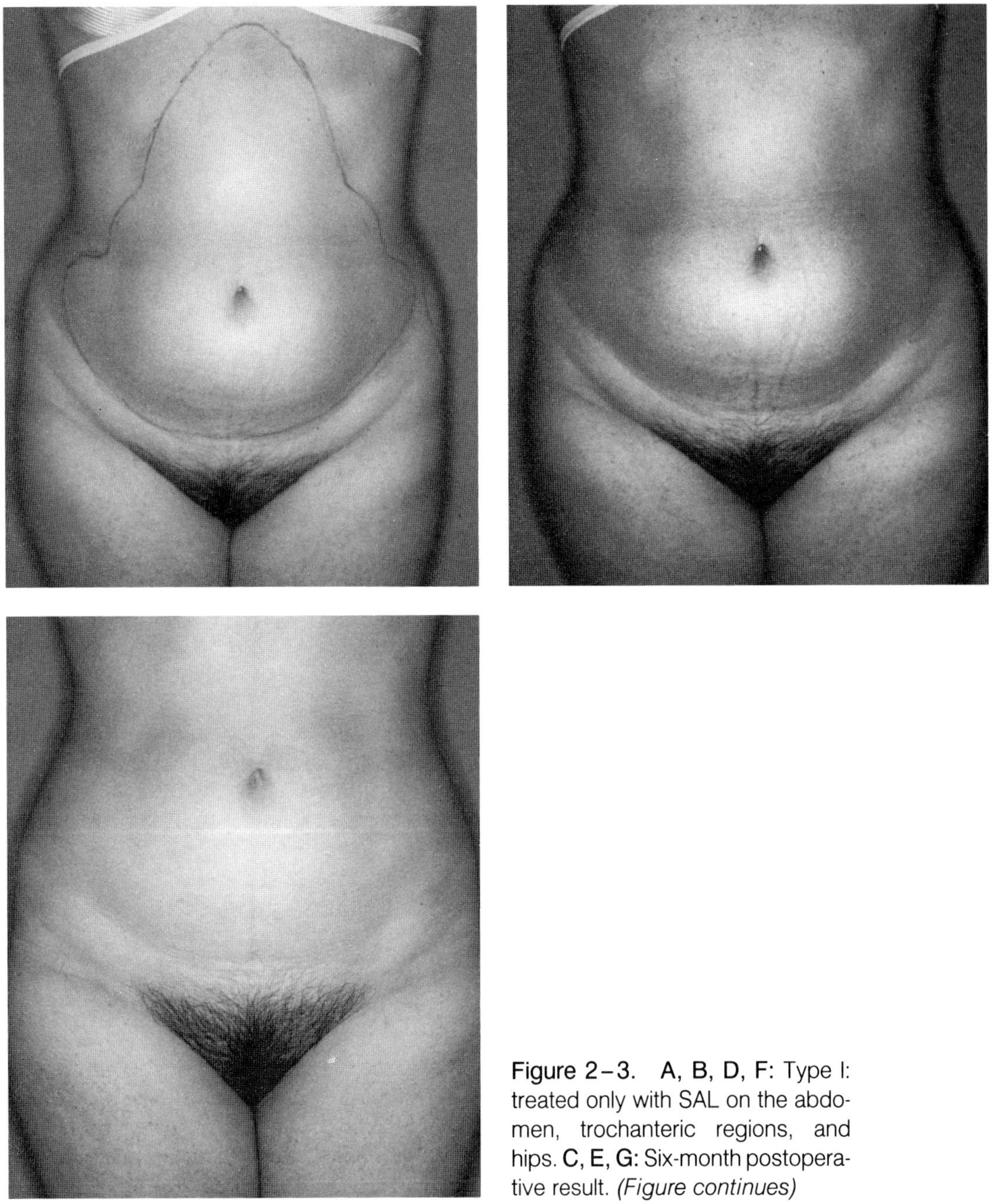

Figure 2–3. A, B, D, F: Type I: treated only with SAL on the abdomen, trochanteric regions, and hips. C, E, G: Six-month postoperative result. *(Figure continues)*

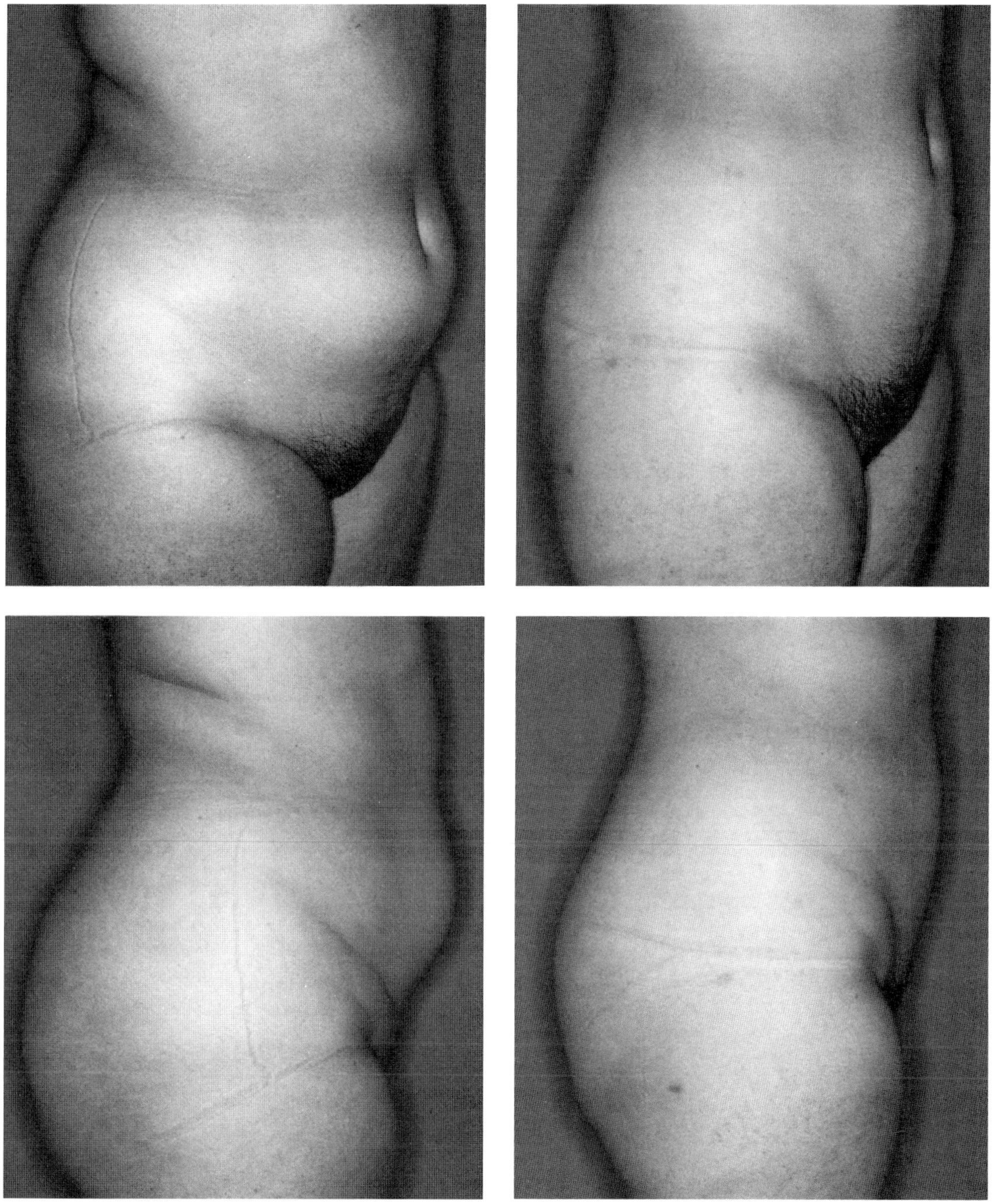

D E F G

Figure 2–3. *(continued)*

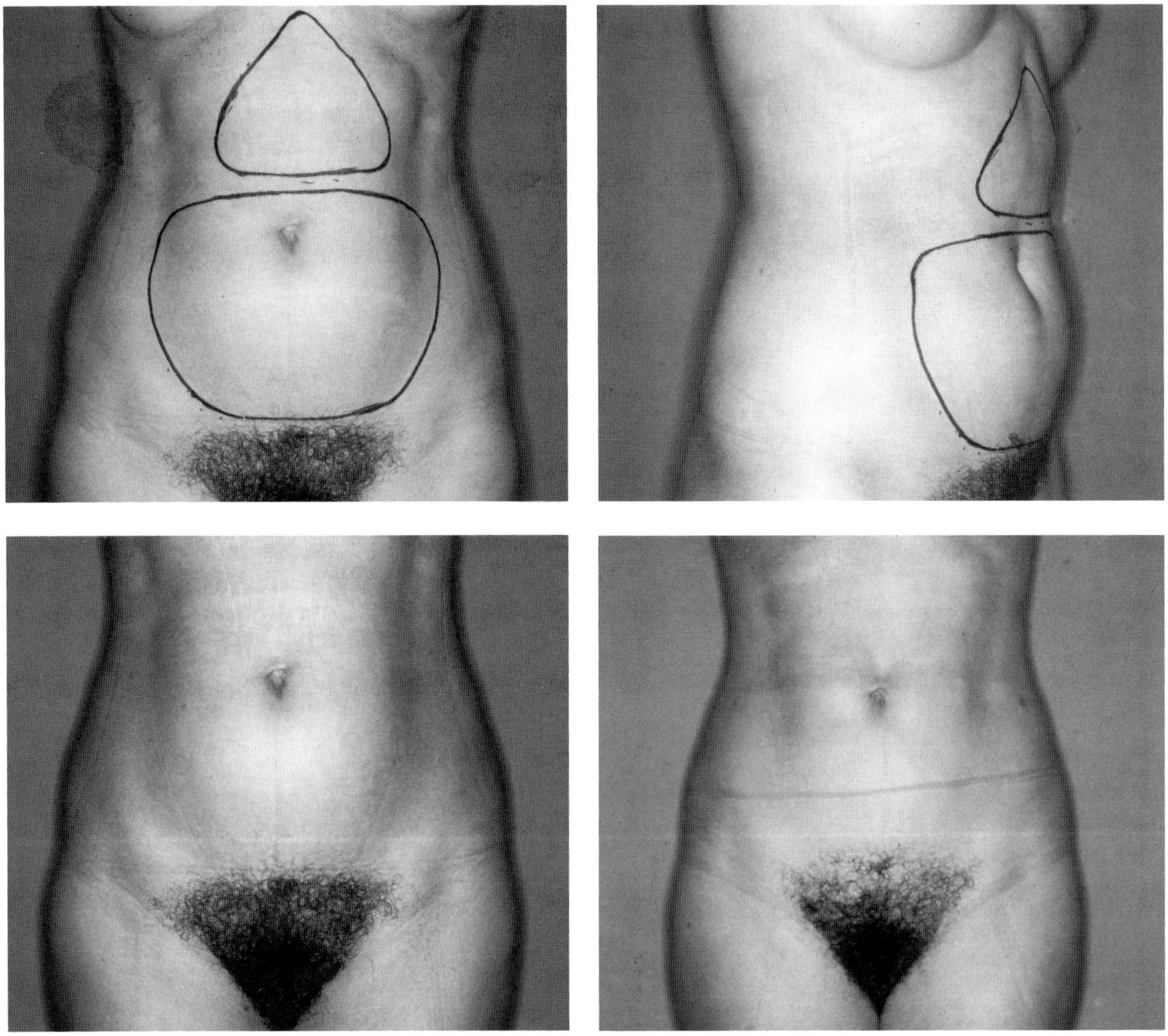

A B C D

Figure 2–4. **A, B, C, E, G:** Type I: treated only with SAL on the upper and lower abdomen. **D, F, H:** Four-month postoperative result. *(Figure continues)*

sisted lipectomy (SAL). This technique is used with one incision in the pubic area to introduce the cannula to reduce the fat in the lower abdomen, in the waist, and to design the semilunar sulcus; a small incision in the margin of the navel is used to introduce the cannula to reduce the fat in the upper abdomen and to design the depression in the middle line. With the use of the tunnel tracer and guided cannulas the incision for SAL may be made in the flanks. To reduce the fat located at the hips, the patient may be maintained in the dorsal position if the adipose deposits do not extend beyond the middle axillary line. If these deposits extend more posteriorly, it is convenient to perform the SAL with the patient in the prone position.

The diameter of the conventional cannulas for SAL in the abdomen is 5 mm, whereas for the guided cannulas it is 8 mm for the abdomen and 6 and 8 mm for the hips.

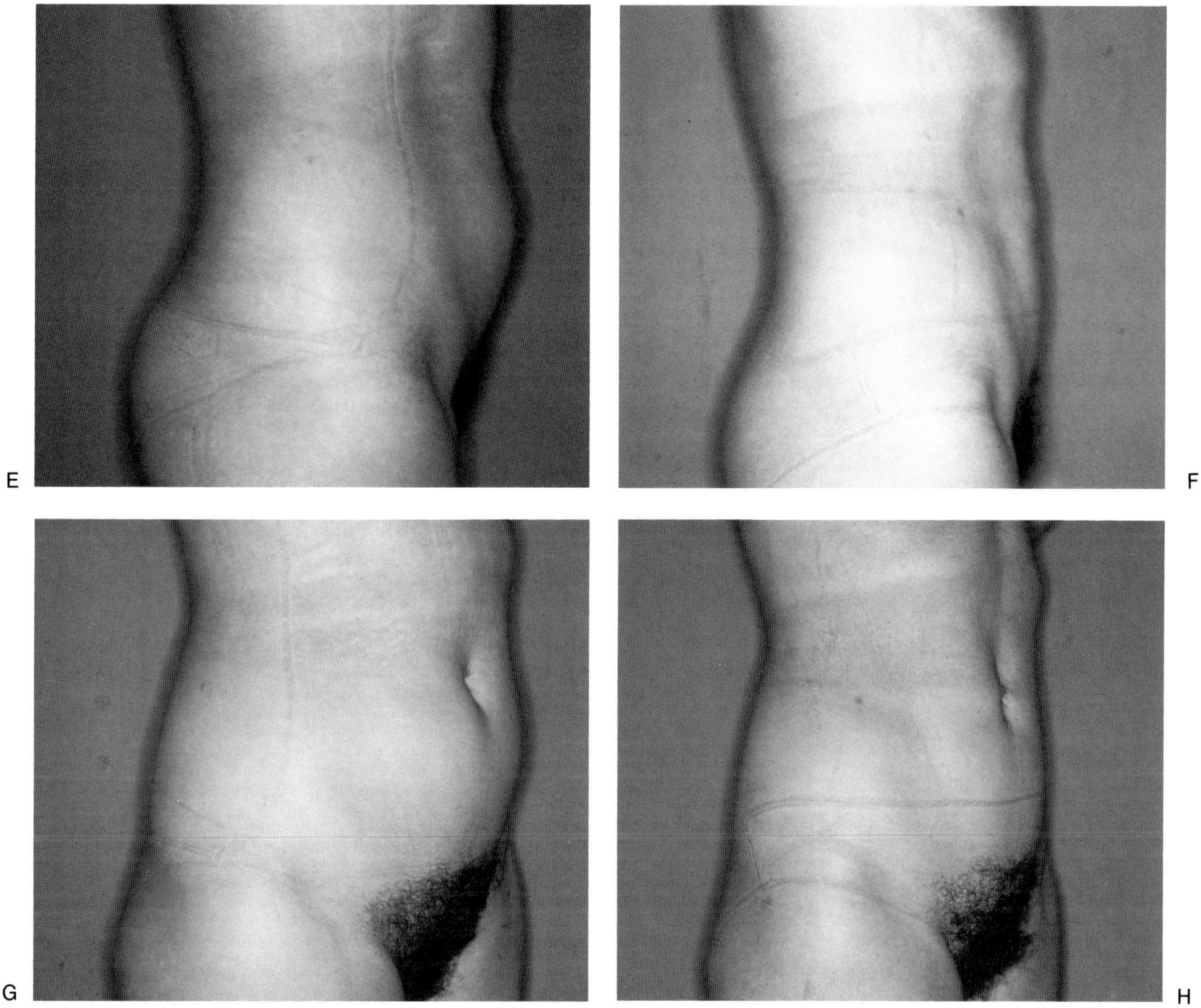

Figure 2–4. *(continued)*

Type II

Patients without laxity of the musculoaponeurotic layer and with mild skin excess in the lower abdomen make up this group. In some, but not all cases, there is an excess of fat in the infraumbilical area (Fig. 2–5A–D). Treatment is performed by a short transverse abdominal incision variable in extension but generally extending only to the inguinal crease. The skin is undermined up to the level of the umbilicus in the midline and 10 cm laterally above it. Open SAL with 5 mm cannula reduces the thickness of the subcutaneous tissue, especially in the waist, in the upper abdomen at the midline to design the medial sulcus, and in the external margin of the rectus muscle to sculpture the depression of the semilunar sulcus. An elliptical area of skin and subcutaneous tissue is resected. The width varies in each case, but usually it does not exceed 8 cm. The flap is defatted up to the area of the umbilicus. A second choice is first to perform SAL and than do the incision and the flap under-

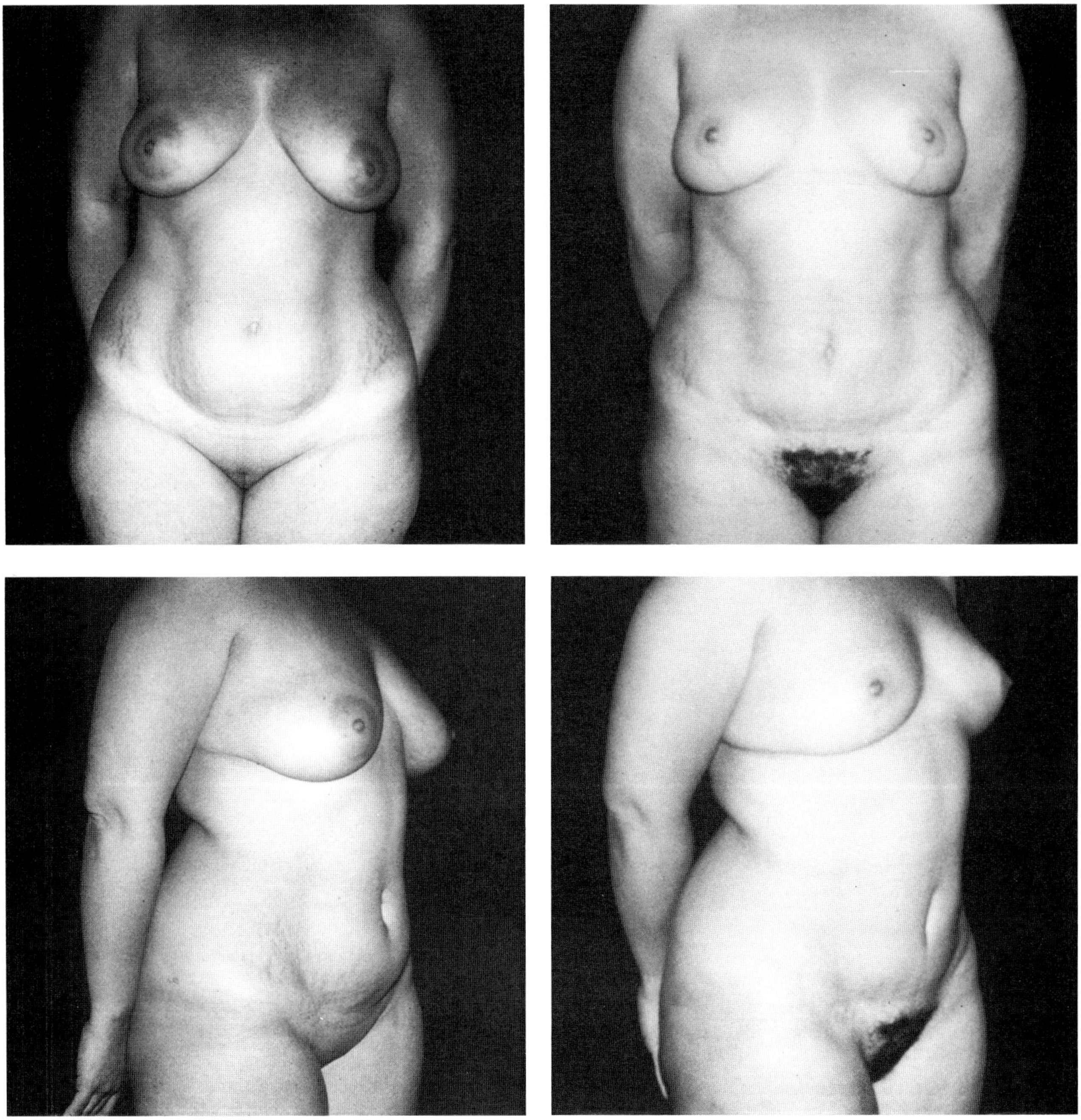

A B

C D

Figure 2–5. **A, C:** Type II: treated with mild cutaneous resection, defatting and suction-assisted lipectomy. **B, D:** One-year postoperative result.

mining; the dissection of the flap is faster and easy. The wound is closed from the lateral side to the midline, distributing the excess skin of the superior flap little by little to avoid "dog-ears" and a long scar.

Type III

These patients are similar to those of type II, but with laxity of the musculoaponeurotic layer in the infraumbilical area (Fig. 2–6A–F). In general,

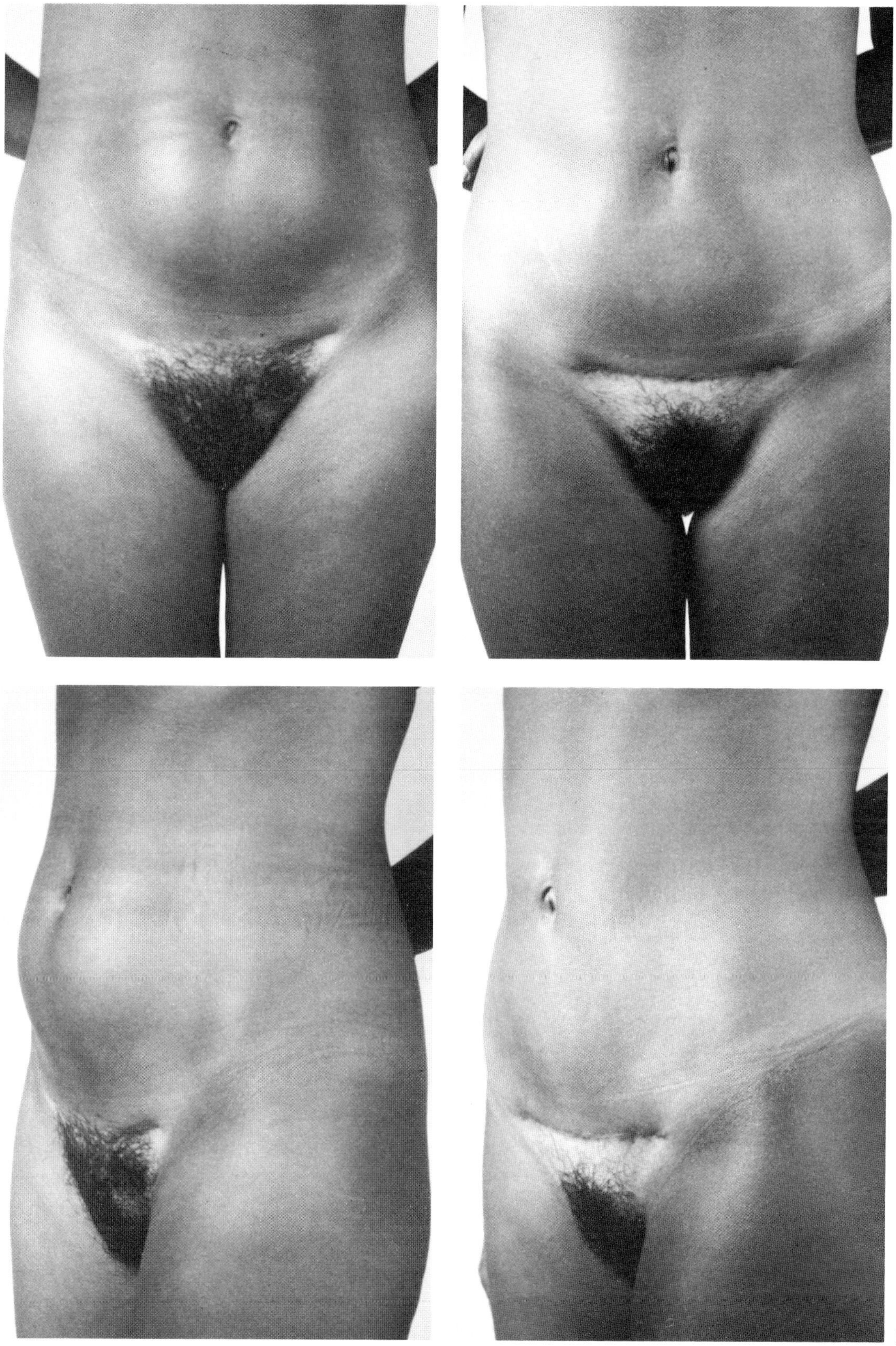

A B C D

Figure 2–6. A, C, E: Type III: treated with mild cutaneous resection, plication of the aponeurosis of the rectus sheath from the umbilicus to the pubis, and suction-assisted lipectomy. B, D, F: Five-month postoperative result. *(Figure continues)*

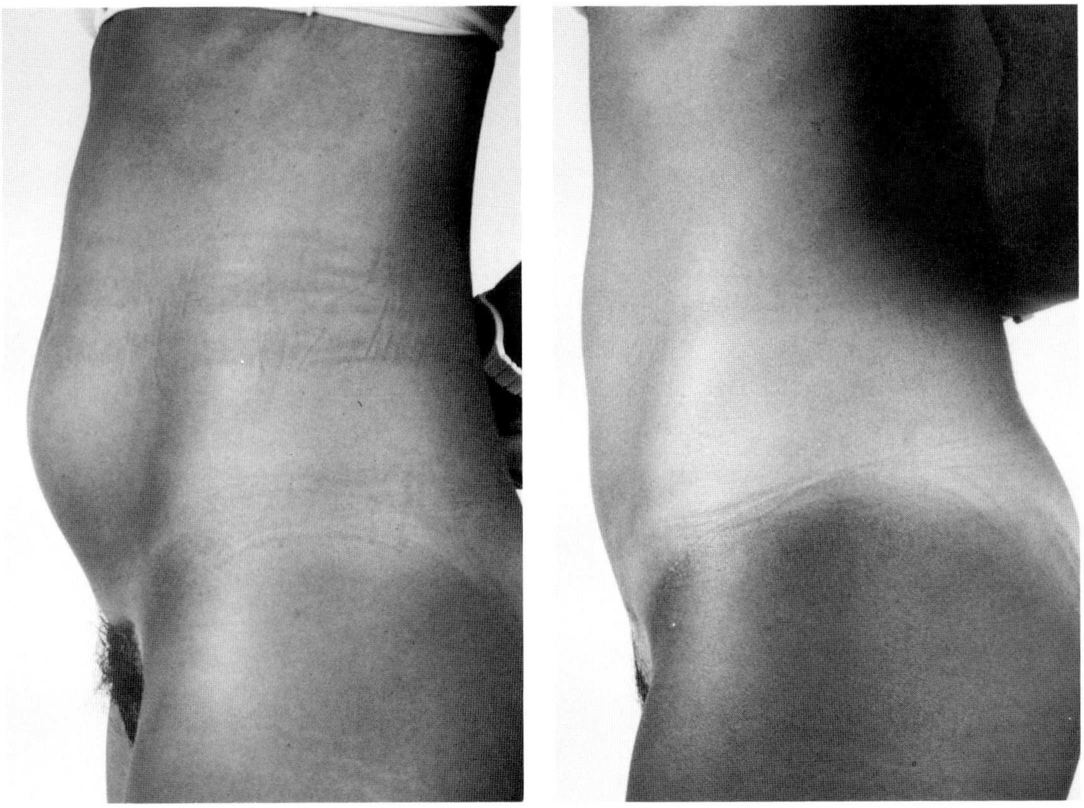

Figure 2–6. *(continued)*

these are patients with one or two previous pregnancies or sedentary nulliparous patients. Treatment is similar to type II, but we include the suture of the rectus diastasis from the pubis to the umbilicus area. The oblique muscle may be disected to reduce the waist if indicated.

Type IV

Patients of this type display a mild excess of skin, various amounts of adipose tissue, and laxity of the musculoaponeurotic system from the xiphoid to the pubis (Fig. 2–7A–D). We include in this group those with the umbilicus more than 14 cm above the pubic symphysis. Treatment consists of skin resection as in types II and III, and subcutaneous defatting. The flap is undermined superiorly up to the xiphoid and to the lower costal margins. The navel can be released (Fig. 2–8A–E) or not (Fig. 2–9A–I) from its insertion on the aponeurosis to allow the treatment of the musculoaponeurotic laxity that is corrected by disecting the rectus muscle and extended oblique diastasis.

Type V

Large amounts of excess skin, varying amounts of adipose tissue, diastasis, and weakness of the entire musculoaponeurotic system are the common characteristics of Type V patients (Fig. 2–10A–F and 2–11A–F). For patients with large excess of skin in the upper abdomen, we use the traditional abdominoplasty or the reverse abdominoplasty technique (type VI). Plication of the musculoaponeurotic system, the rectii, and the external oblique muscles is similar to that done in type IV.

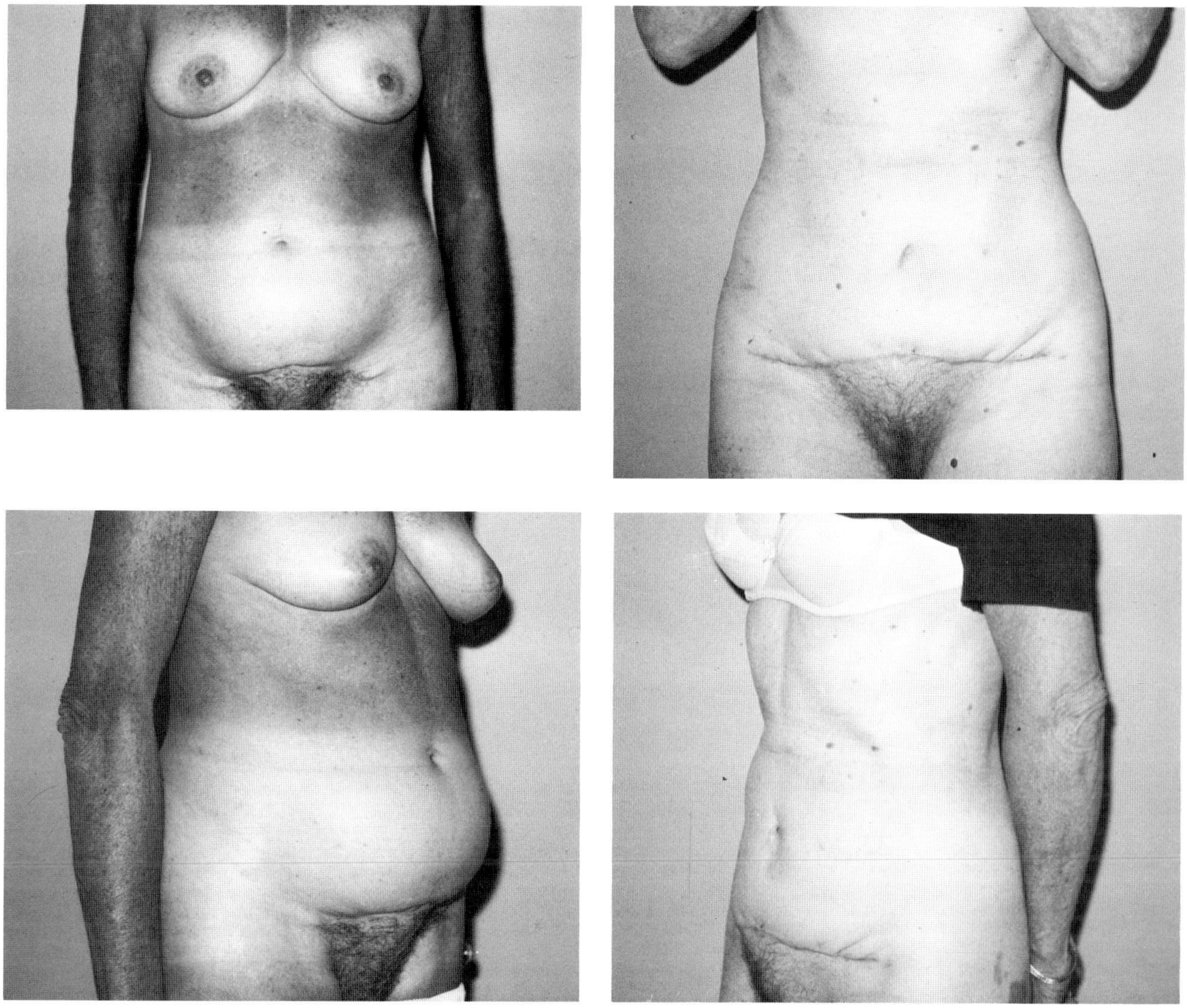

Figure 2–7. A, C: Type IV: great laxity of the musculoaponeurotic layer treated with mild cutaneous resection and repositioning and plication of the rectus sheath and advancement of the external oblique muscles. The stalk was released from its insertion and reinserted 2 cm below its original position. B, D: Postoperative result at 1 year.

Type VI

Large amounts of excess skin only or preferably in the supraumbilical region is one of the determining factors of patients who fit into this category. They also need a breast lifting, breast augmentation, or breast reduction, or they have a scar from a previous mammoplasty. Incision in the mammary sulcus that joins in the middle line is also necessary. After dissection of the flap up to the navel and laterally a little lower, the flap is superiorly extended and the excess is removed following the mammary sulcus (Figs. 2–12A–D, 2–13A–D).

If breast augmentation is needed, part of the flap is deepithelized and fixed to the pectoralis fascia. Plicature of the rectus muscles is performed only exceptionally.

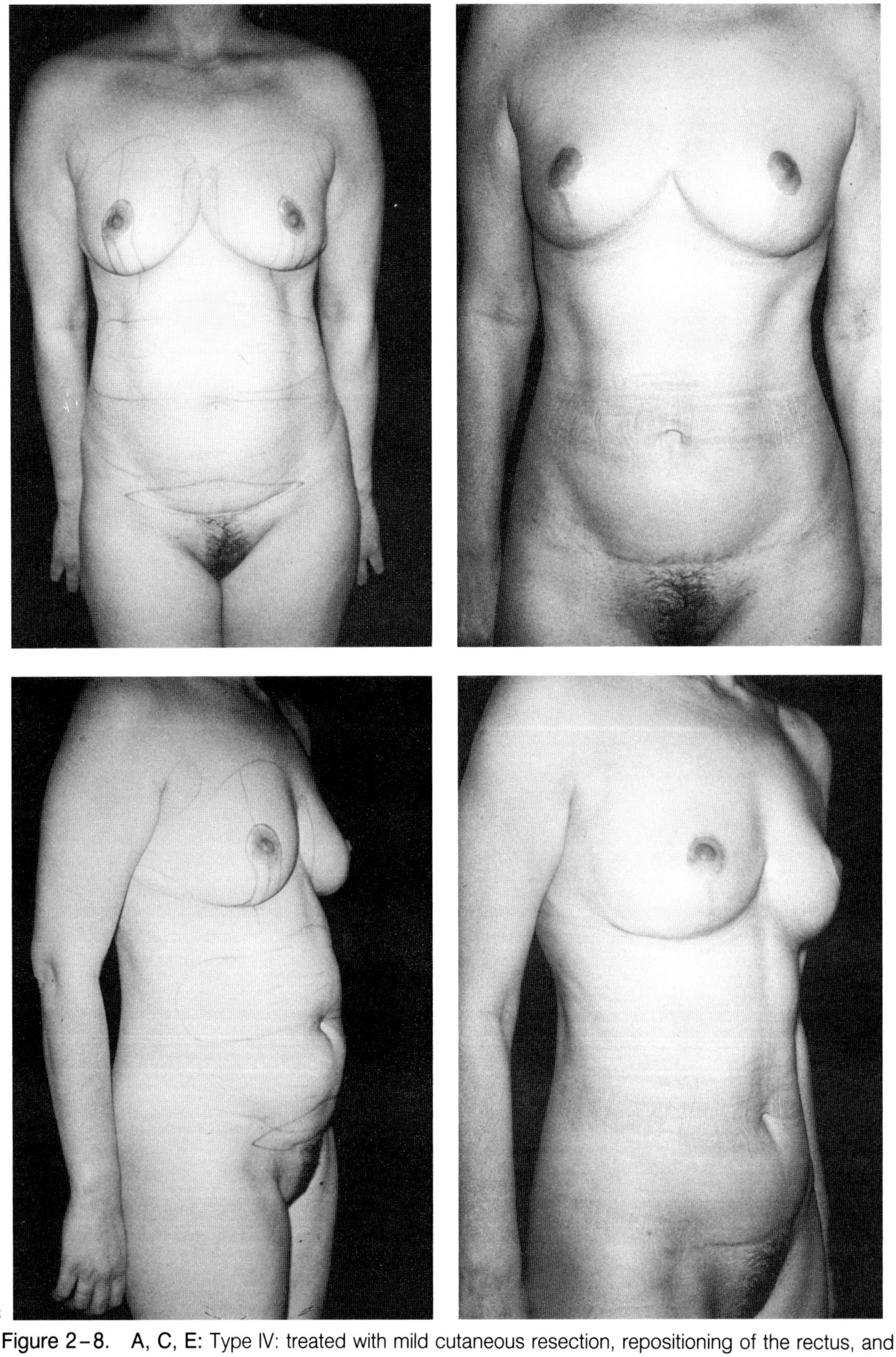

A B

C D

Figure 2–8. **A, C, E:** Type IV: treated with mild cutaneous resection, repositioning of the rectus, and advancement of the external oblique muscles and suction-assisted lipectomy. The navel was released from its insertion and reinserted in the original position (see Fig. 3–13). **B, D, F:** Postoperative result at 1 year. *(Figure continues)*

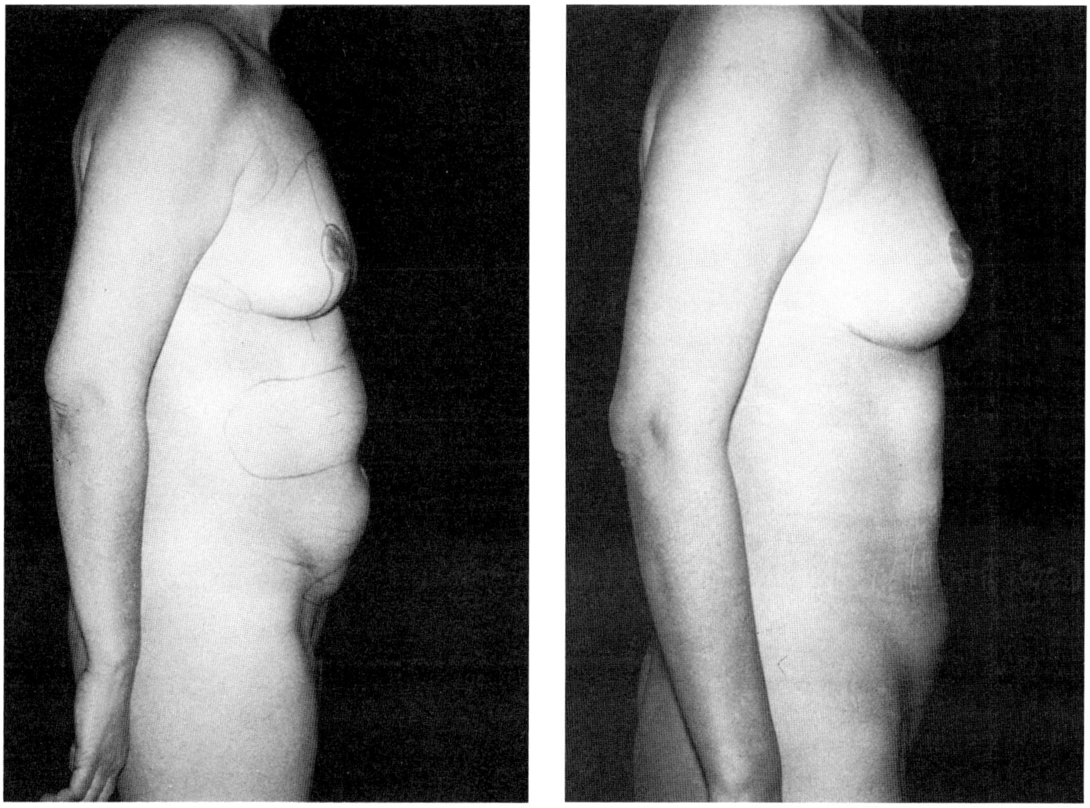

E F

Figure 2–8. *(continued)*

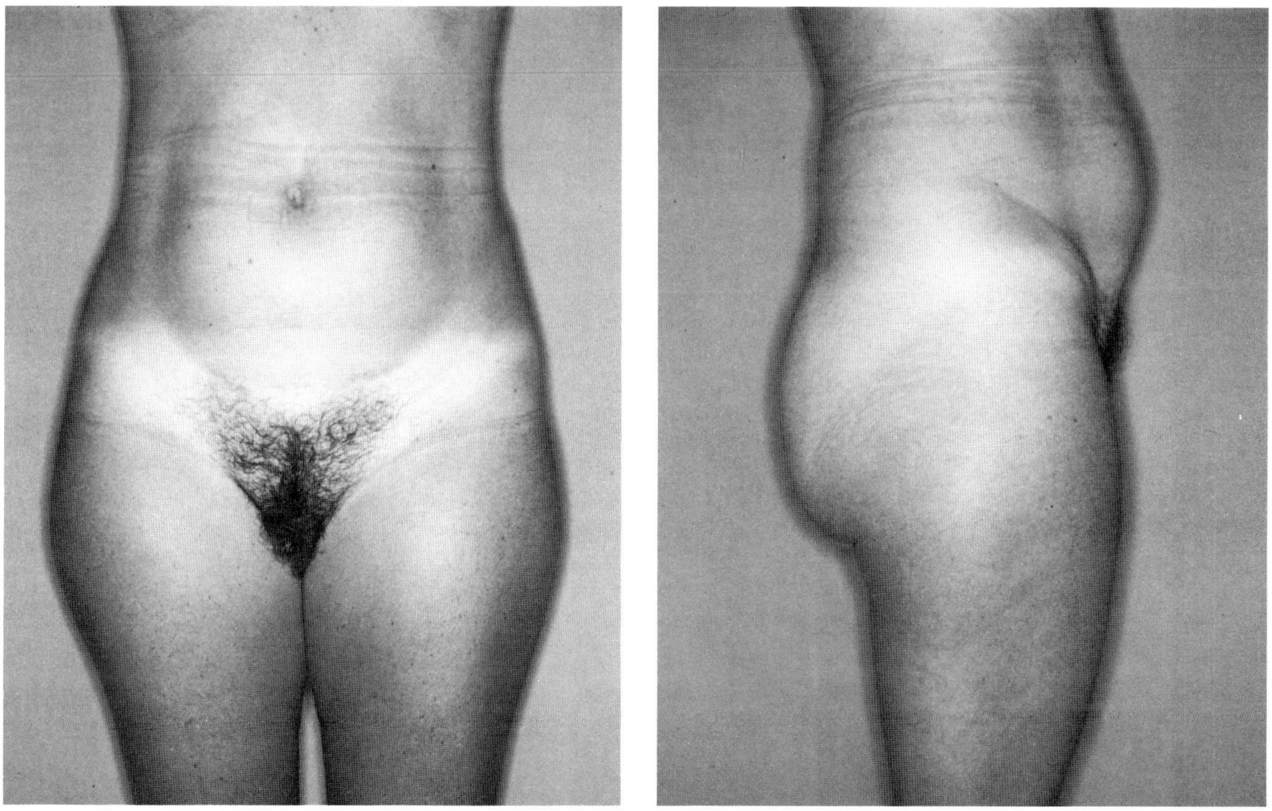

A B

Figure 2–9. **A, B**: Type IV: treated with mild cutaneous resection, SAL, plication of the rectus muscles from the xiphoid to the pubis without releasing the navel (see Fig. 3–14). **C, D**: Postoperative result after 2 months. *(Figure continues)*

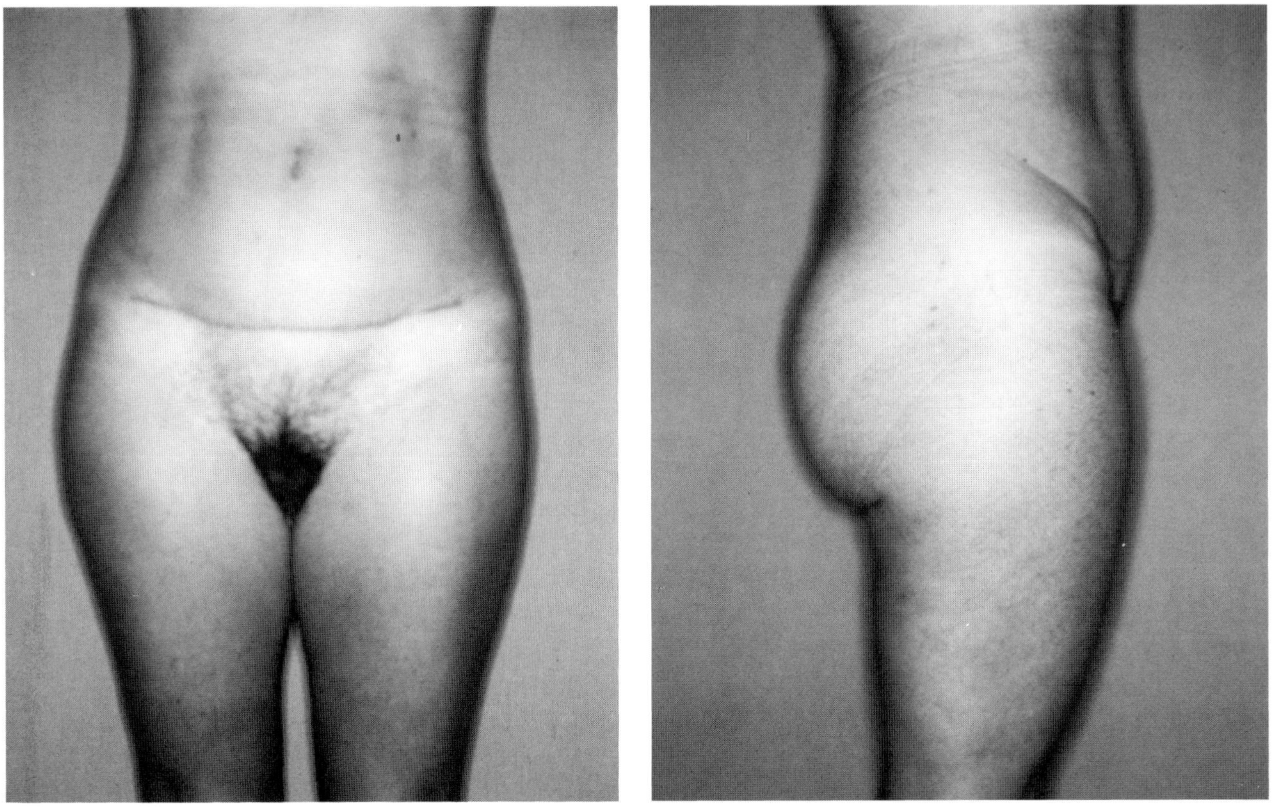

C D

Figure 2–9. *(continued)*

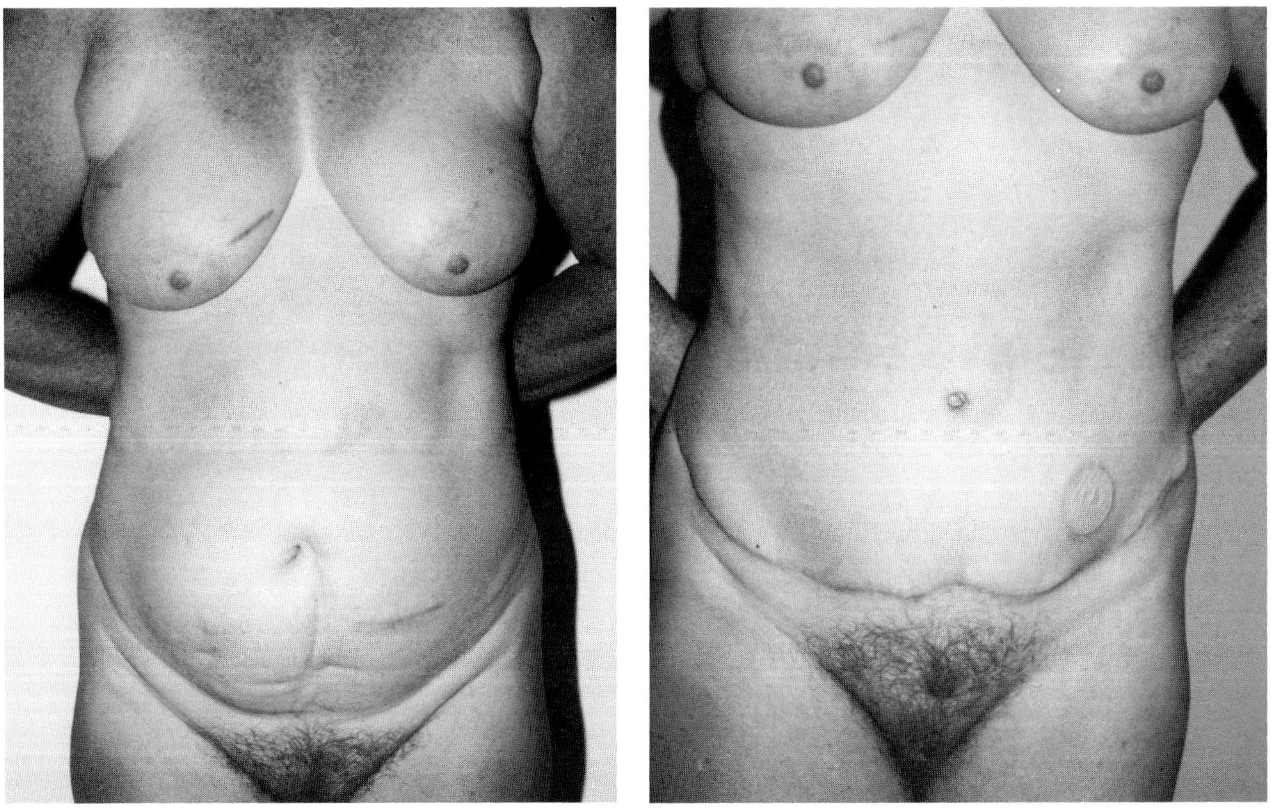

A B

Figure 2–10. **A, C, E:** Type V: cutaneous resection from the pubis to the umbilicus; plicature of the rectus sheath and advancement of the external oblique muscles, defatting of the flap with the knife to rebuild the "lyre," and suction-assisted lipectomy in the waist and hips. **B, D, F:** Six-month postoperative result.

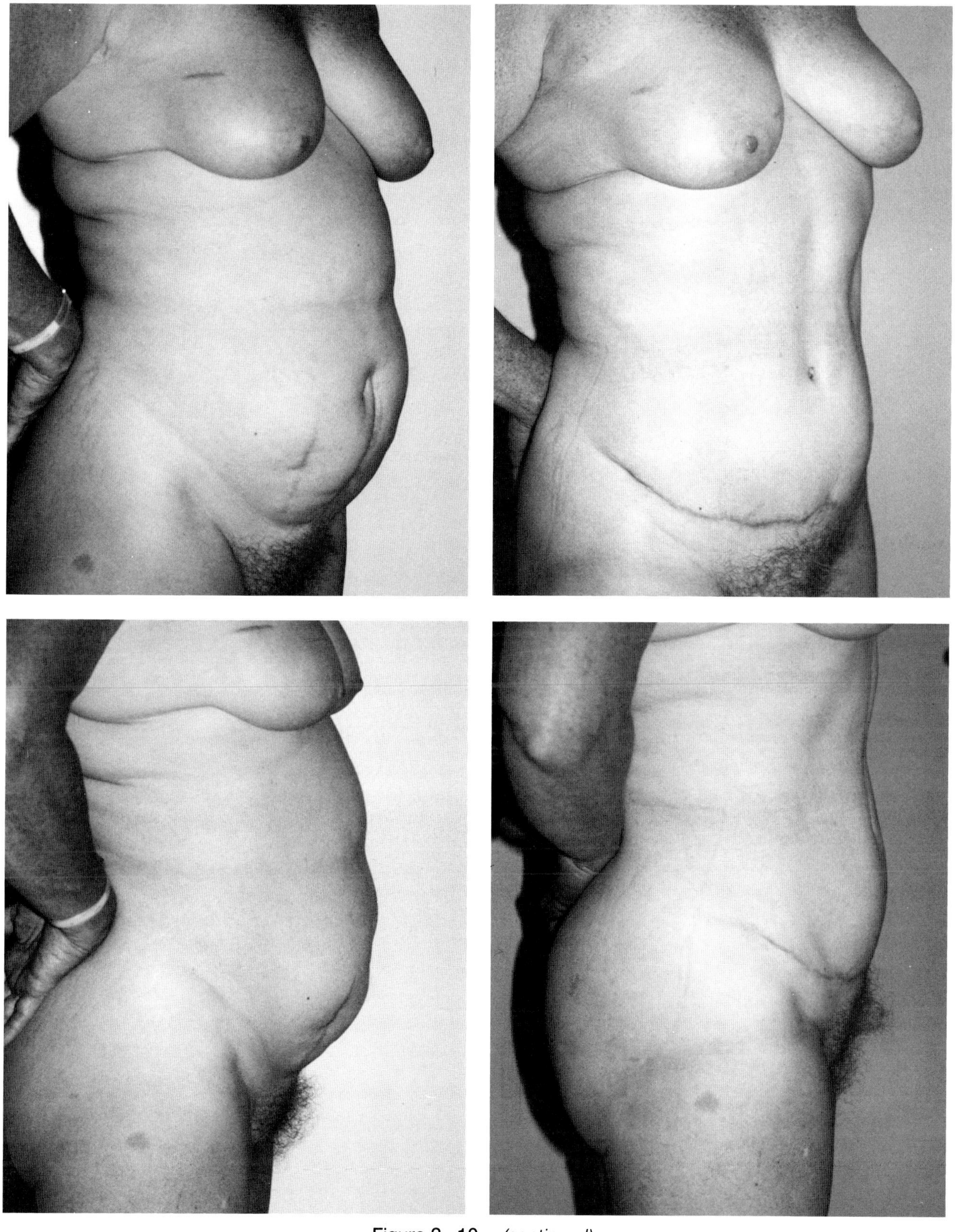

C D E F

Figure 2–10. *(continued)*

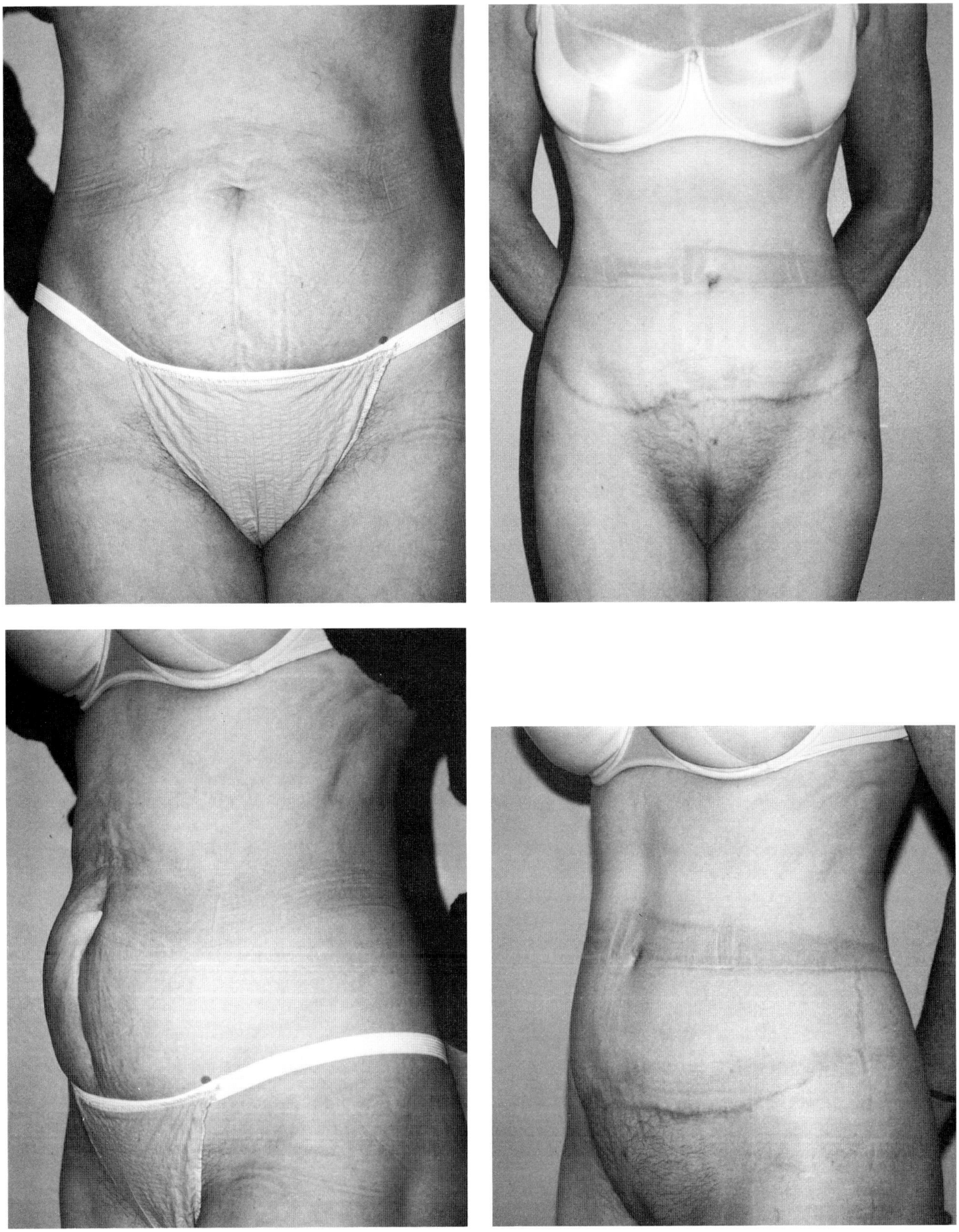

A B C D

Figure 2–11. **A, C, E:** Type V: treated with cutaneous resection of skin from the pubis to the umbilicus; plication of the rectus sheath from xiphoid to the pubis and advancement of the external oblique muscles; defatting of the flap with the knife to reshape the abdominal lyre. **B, D, F:** Eight-month postoperative result. *(Figure continues)*

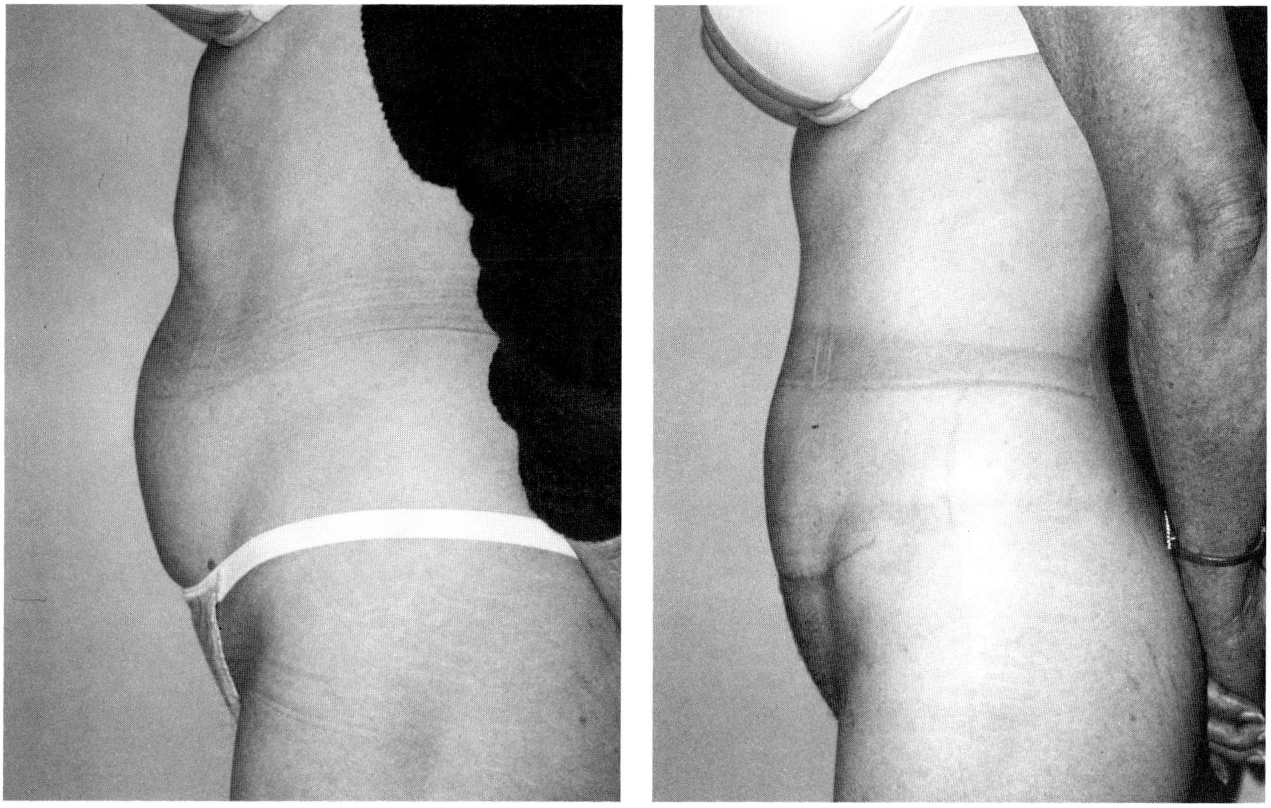

E F

Figure 2–11. *(continued)*

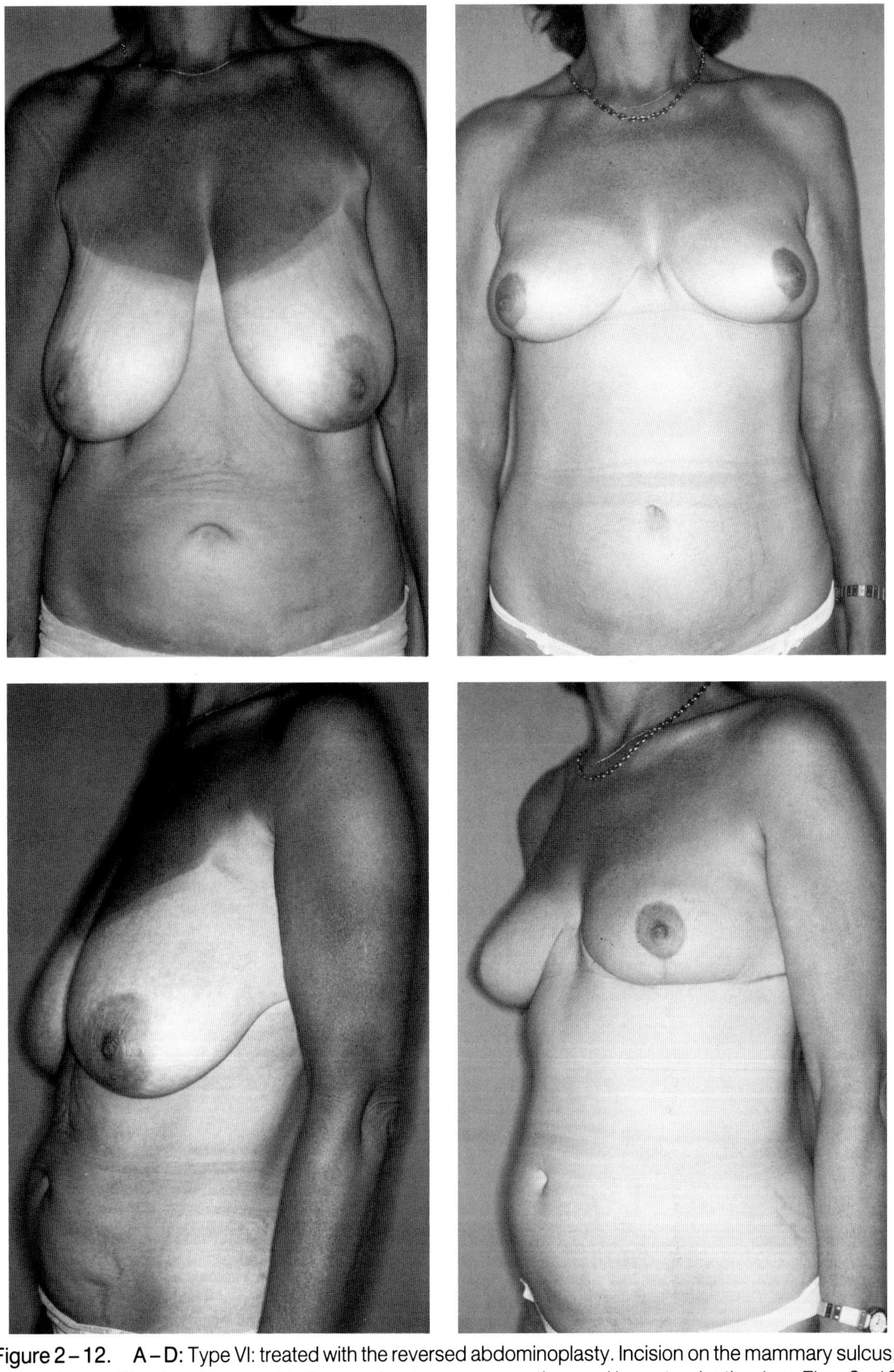

A B C D

Figure 2–12. A–D: Type VI: treated with the reversed abdominoplasty. Incision on the mammary sulcus, undermining of the flap downward to the navel, cutaneous resection, and breast reduction (see Figs. 3–16 and 3–46).

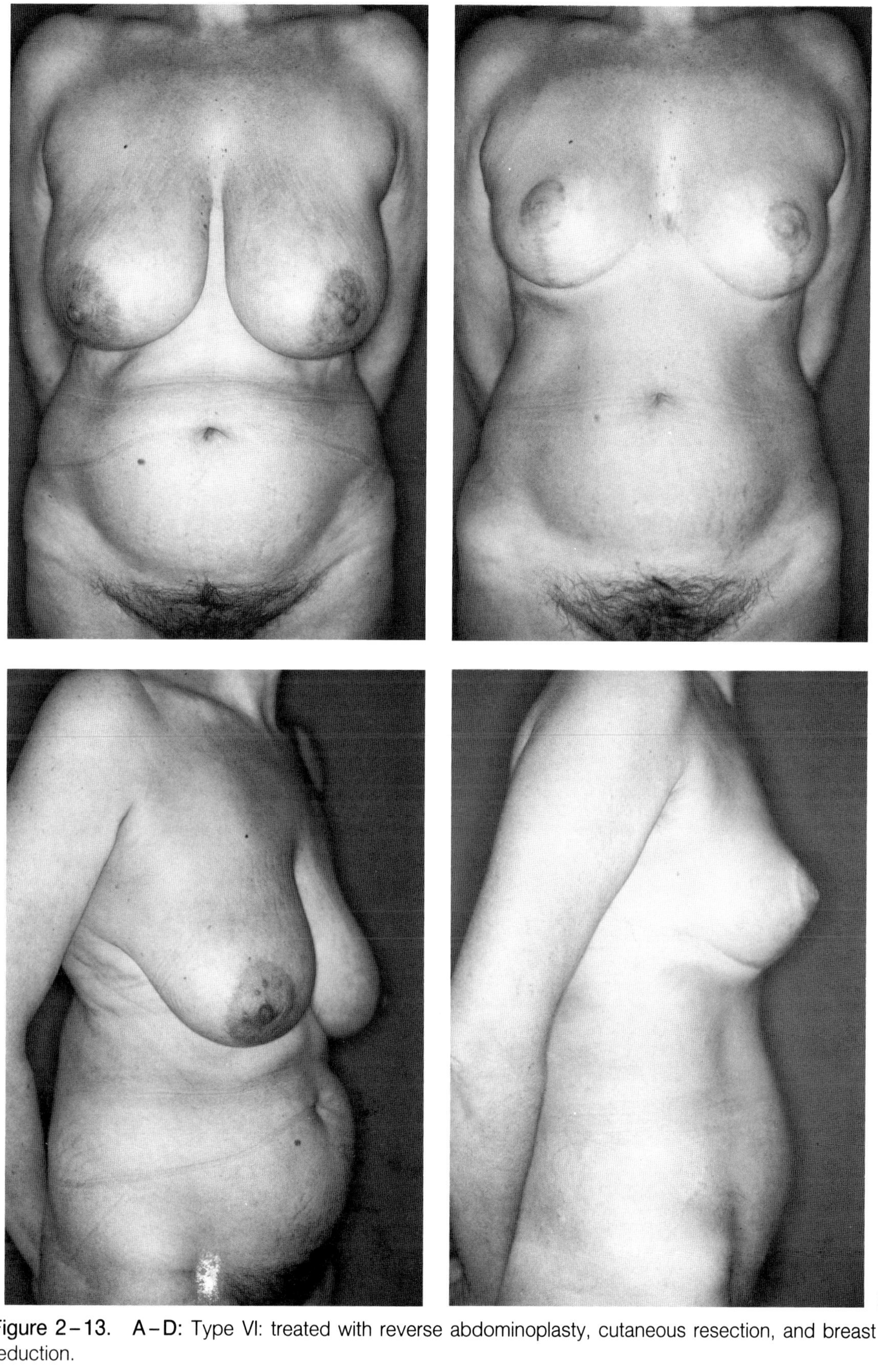

A B C D

Figure 2–13. A–D: Type VI: treated with reverse abdominoplasty, cutaneous resection, and breast reduction.

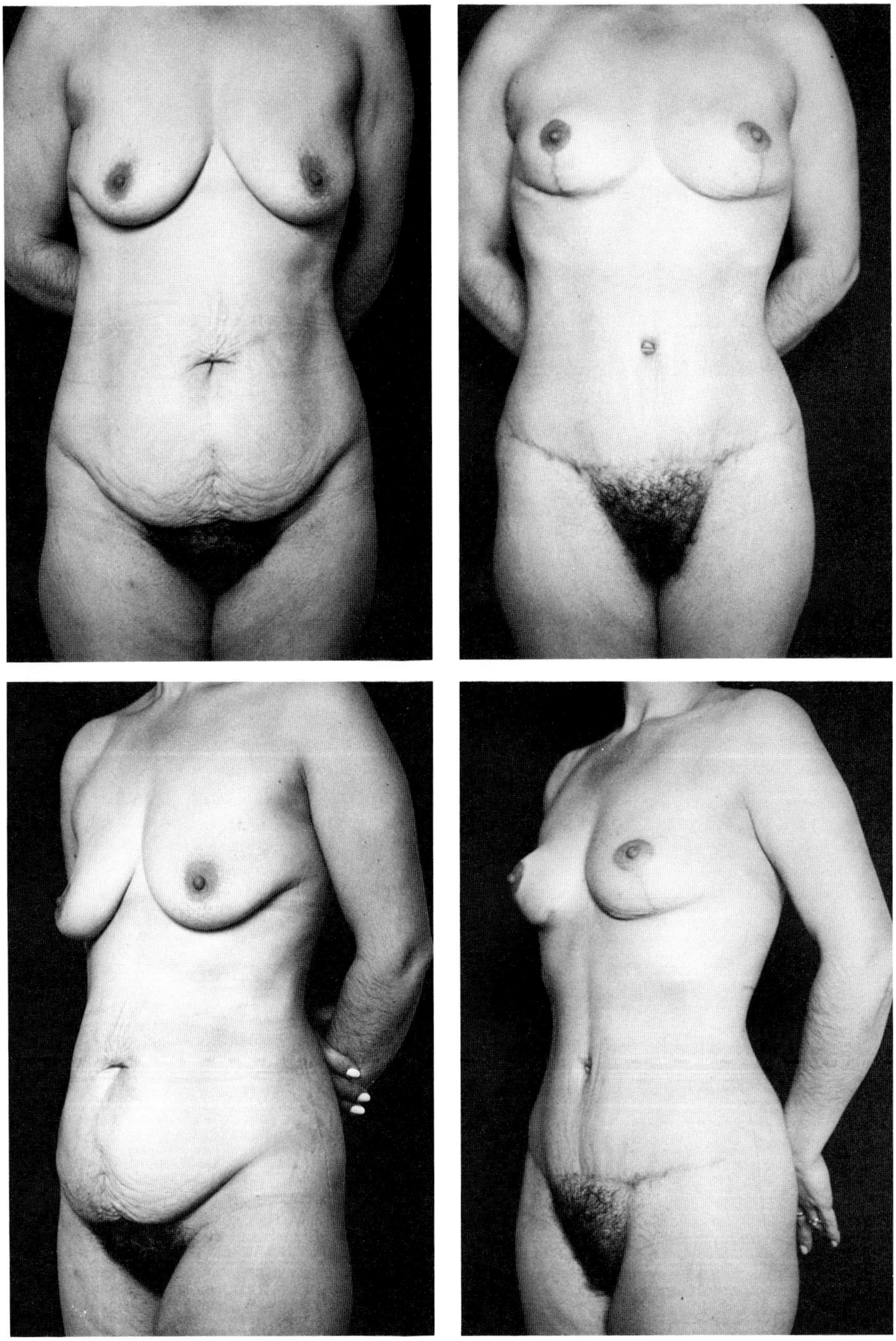

A B

C D

Figure 2–14. A–F: A very common combination of procedures: breast reduction and abdominoplasty. The breast was treated with the traditional inverted "T" procedure. The abdomen was treated as described for the type V abdomen.

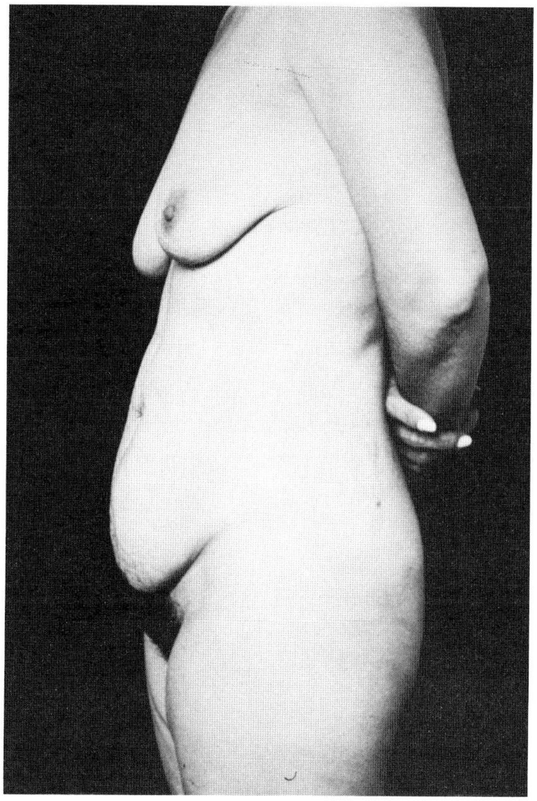

E

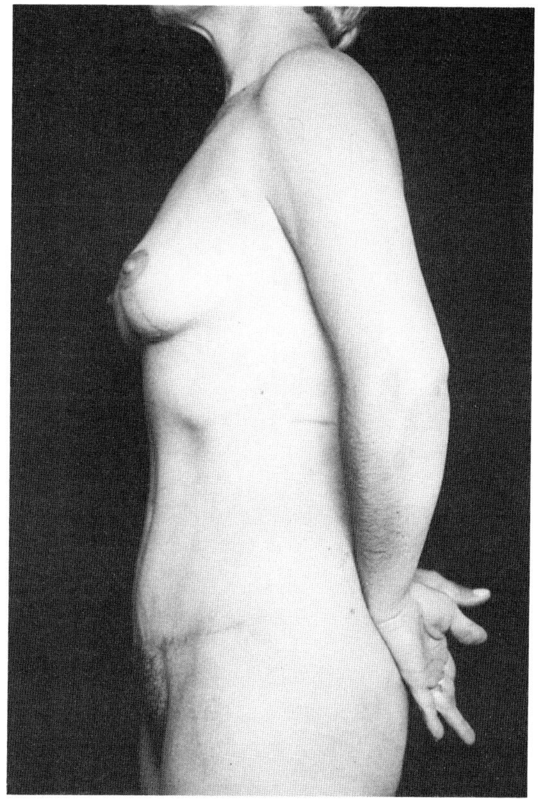

F

Figure 2–14. *(continued)*

COMBINED AESTHETIC PROCEDURES

During consultation, it is common for the patient to request treatment of other areas, such as the breasts, gluteotrochanteric region, thighs, knees, and arms. Less frequently, the patient asks for a face-lift. Naturally, undertaking these combined surgeries will depend on the experience of the surgeon and his team, the health of the patient, and the evaluation of all risk factors (Fig. 2–14A–F).

PATIENT EDUCATION

The patient must be very well informed of all the details of the surgery: risks, time of the operation, results that can be obtained, limitations, size and position of scars, duration, and symptoms of the postoperative period. Among the risks, we must inform the patient of the possibility of seromas, hematomas, infection and necrosis of the flap, and thrombosis. These complications will be discussed in detail in Chapter 4.

The time of surgery depends on the type of abdomen and the experience of the surgeon, but, in general, it will last from 1½ to 3 hours. Naturally, in combined surgeries the times of all of the procedures must be included. Among the immediate postoperative symptoms, the patient must be informed of difficulty in extending the trunk with the abdominal sensation of traction, a certain amount of pain with movements, abdominal distension caused by gas (it is recommended that gas relief medications be prescribed in the postoperative period), and absence of sensation in the infraumbilical area for a period of 3 months.

Overweight patients are requested to make an effort to lose as much weight as they can. A program of losing weight preoperatively and loss of weight in the postoperative period is established with our psychological support and with the help of an endocrinologist and a program of exercises.

3

Operative Technique

IMMEDIATE PREOPERATIVE ROUTINE

The patient undergoes routine clinical and laboratory examinations. Blood tests and a clinical preoperative examination are important. A specific cardiovascular history and examinations are also obtained. In patients with preoperative history of phlebitis special care has to be taken during surgery. The patient is asked to suspend any medications being taken for 48 hours before surgery. Aspirin and anticontraceptive agents are to be suspended 2 weeks prior to surgery. Patients who are heavy cigarette smokers must be intensively warned not to smoke 2 weeks prior to surgery.

The incision can be previously marked with the patient standing up and wearing a bikini to be sure that the scar will be covered or it can be marked when the patient is lying down on the operating table. Preparation and antisepsis are done from the breasts to the superior third of the thighs and from one posterior axillary line to the other.

The patient is placed in the dorsal position and the upper part of the trunk is slightly elevated, with the arms at a 90° angle from the body.

ANESTHESIA

All the operations are performed under general anesthesia with hypotension. Epidural anesthesia can also be used by an experienced team.

The use of anesthesia with hypotension is not new in plastic surgery, since it was used by McIndoe in 1956. The technique reduces the surgical time and the loss of blood, and a clean field permits the surgeon to work better and more precisely.

We have been using hypotension since 1967 in abdominoplasty as well as more recently with suction-assisted lipectomy (SAL). Since the blood loss is widely reduced, we can combine other procedures, such as mammaplasty and blepharoplasty. The need for blood transfusion is dramatically reduced with hypotension. When the surgeon is performing the incision and dissection, the blood systolic pressure is maintained between 70 and 85 mmHg and is increased to 90 to 95 mmHg after this period. When we are doing only SAL, it is recommended that the blood pressure be maintained constantly between 70 and 75 mmHg during the period of the operation until the dressing is applied.

LIPOSUCTION

Before we use SAL in the abdomen, we need to keep in mind the following:

- The absence of homogeneity of the thickness of the adipose tissue and the variable difficulty of doing SAL from one area to another.
- The presence of large perforating vessels that in multiparous patients can be very thick, tortuous, and less mobile. The rupture of one of these vessels can produce large blood loss and hematoma.
- The presence of the abdominal cavity, which can be easily perforated, particularly if there are hernias.
- The penetration of the cannulas into the abdominal cavity must be avoided. It is wise to pinch the

cutaneous tissue with the left hand to feel the direction and depth of the movements of the cannulas.

- The tracer and the guided cannulas are best indicated for the abdomen because a more regular liposuction occurs, which is safer because of reduced blood loss and less possibility of penetrating the abdominal cavity. In all, it is less traumatic with faster recovery of the patients.
- When we perform liposuction of the upper abdomen, it is important to extend it over the ribs to avoid the artificial production of a step-like effect.

We begin the operation by marking the areas with a tunnel tracer (Fig. 3–1), which is made of stainless steel bars joined at one end to a handle that permits the bars to turn radially and consequently to open or close like a fan. Silicone crests are attached to the lower edges of the bars so that when coated with surgical ink the tunnels are marked on the abdomen. (Fig. 3–2A, B).

The guide and the cannula (Fig. 3–3A, B) are introduced together, with the orifices facing downward following the direction of each marked line.

Once introduced, the guide remains inside while the cannula is moved evenly, between 15 and 30 strokes, depending on the amount of fat to be aspirated. Without removing the guide, it is turned to the right and between 5 and 20 strokes are made. The cannula is then turned to the left and the same procedure is followed. Homogeneous lipoaspiration among the different tunnels is achieved with these changes of direction (Fig. 3–4A–D). As with liposuction with a conventional cannula, it is recommended that the number of strokes in the marginal areas be reduced and that the length of the penetration by cannula be controlled in order to avoid excessive extraction in peripheral zones and the more proximal ones where the tunnels meet. Generally, crisscross liposuction is recommended and the same procedure should be repeated with the second set of tunnels marked from the selected entrance point. The number of strokes to use depends on the particular case. When the fat is considerably thick or a cannula with a very fine caliber is used, a second more superficial level of aspiration over the entire area or limited to the most prominent zones might be indicated.

We believe that it is extremely useful to record all of the operative data, which, taken together, make up an authentic surgical protocol (Fig. 3–5A, B). Consequently, the purpose of the graphic record is to: help the surgeon in systematizing the technique; act as an accurate account of the details of the technique; be used as a pattern for the opposite area in bilateral cases; collect data in an orderly manner for statistical studies; provide a picture, at a glance, of the data on the operation undertaken.

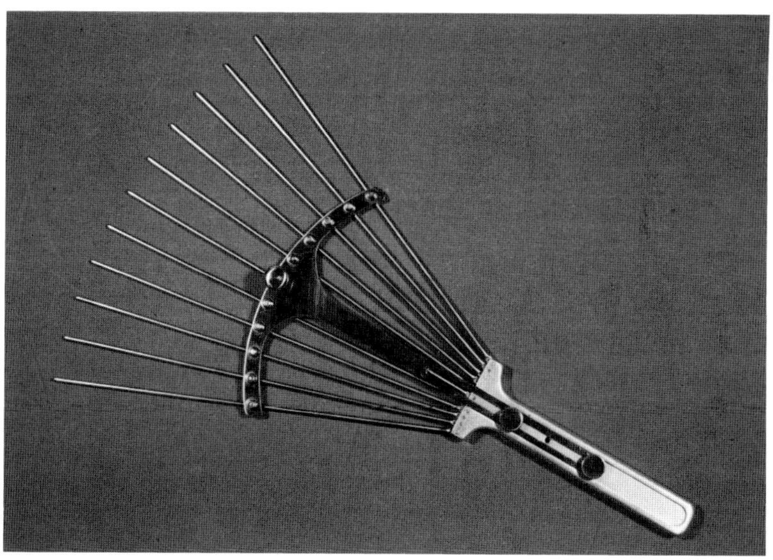

Figure 3–1. Tunnel tracer to mark the tunnels for SAL.

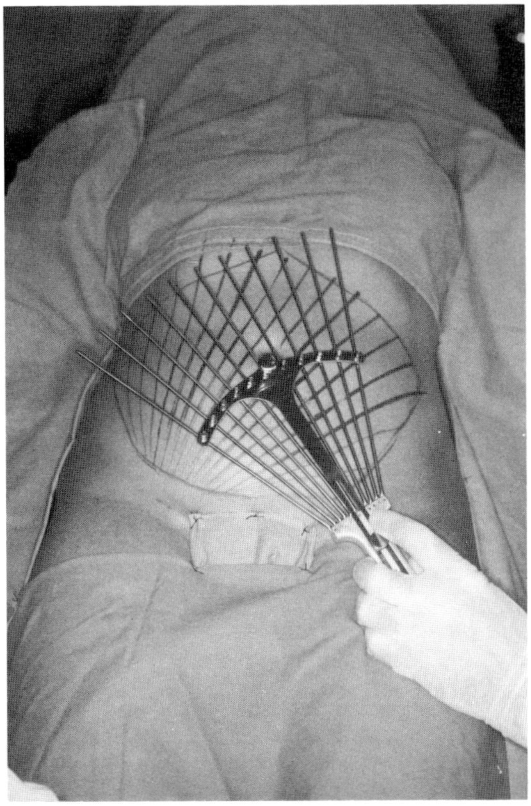
A

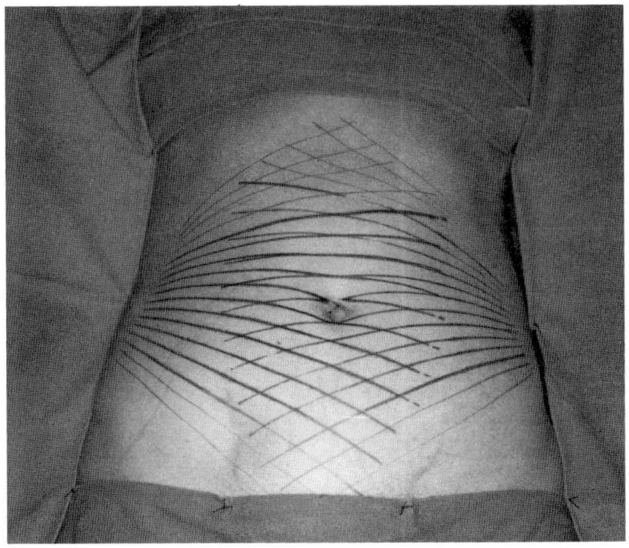
B

Figure 3-2. A, B: The tunnels are marked with surgical ink on the skin.

It should be pointed out that systematizing the technique should not be interpreted as creating a rigid criterion, but rather an ancillary device to help be aware of changes necessary in each case. This is useful, since asymmetries or other morphologic peculiarities exist, suggesting the need for variations in the number of tunnels or cannula strokes or in the extent of the strokes.

Surgery, and particularly plastic surgery, is both a science and an art. Consequently, we cannot sep-

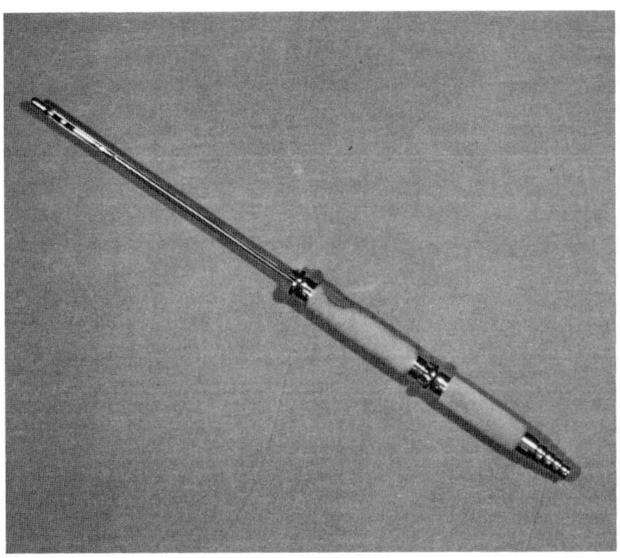
A

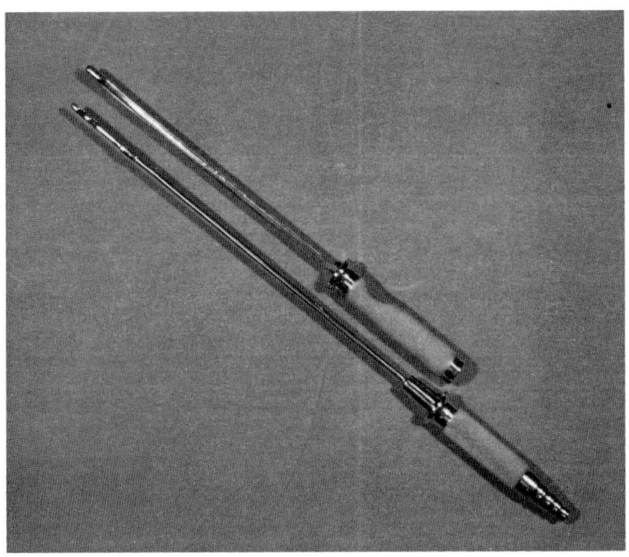
B

Figure 3-3. A, B: The guide and cannula are introduced together for SAL.

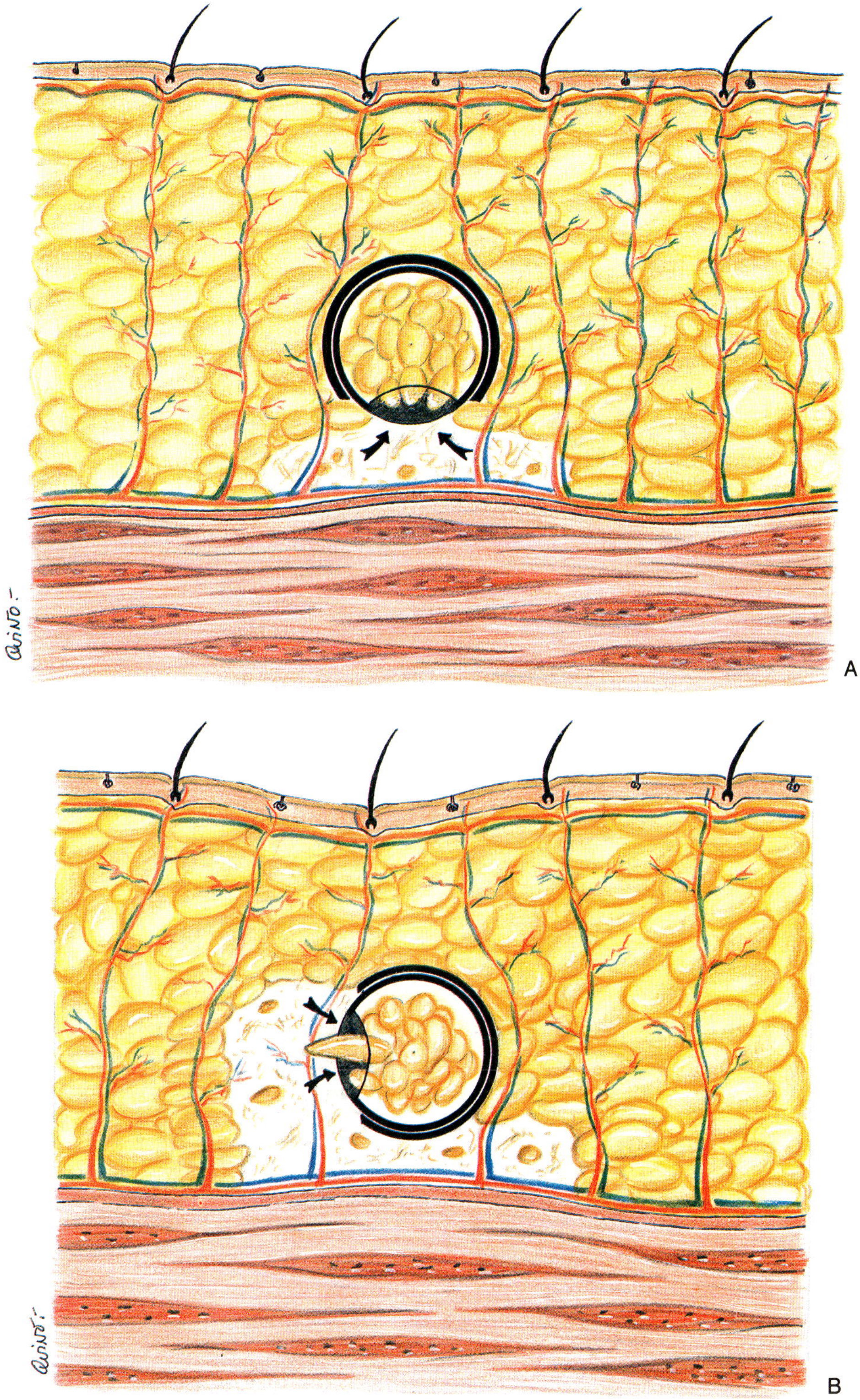

Figure 3–4. A–D: Without removing the guide, the fat is aspirated in all directions. *(Figure continues)*

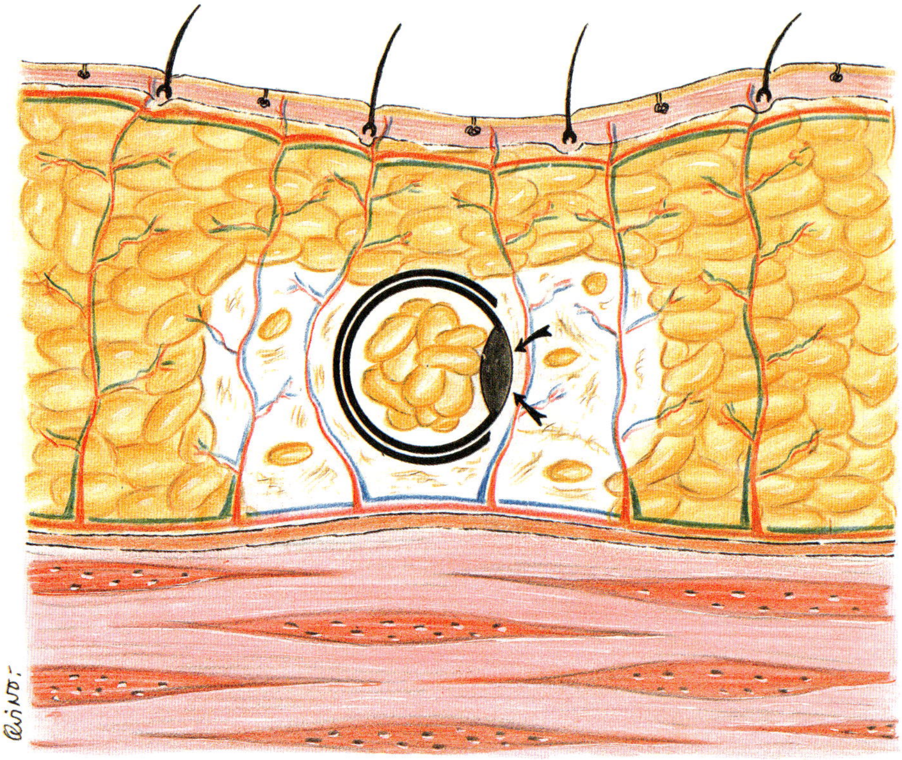

C

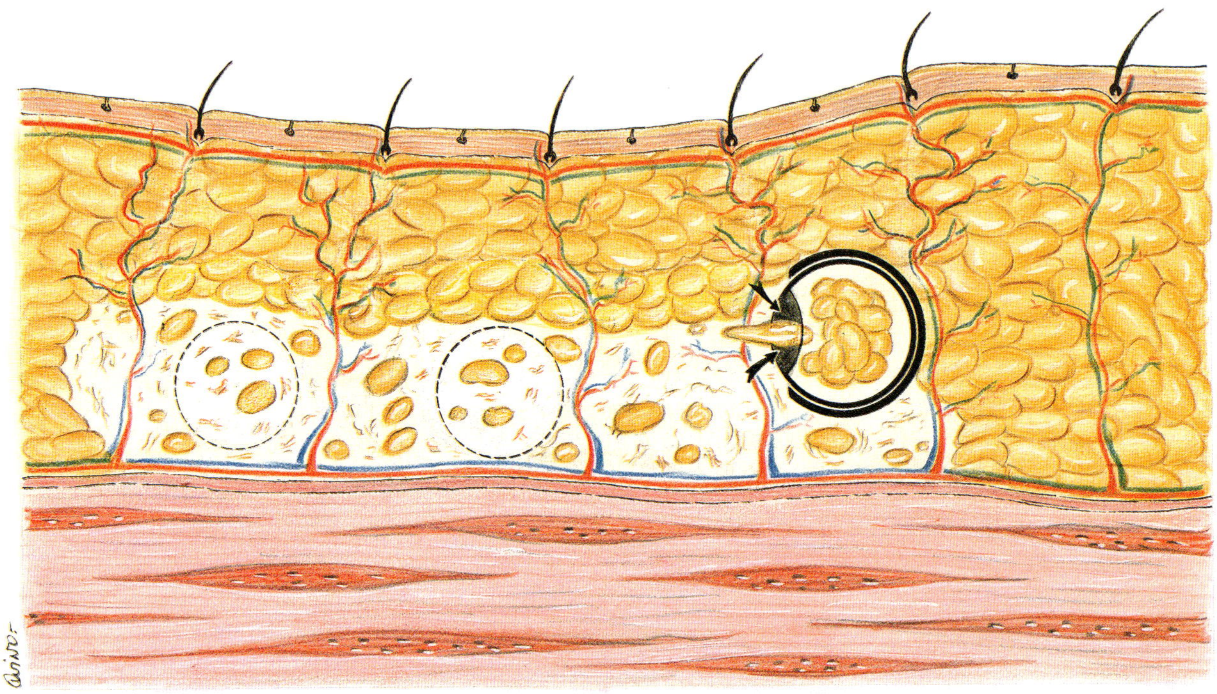

D

Figure 3–4. *(continued)*

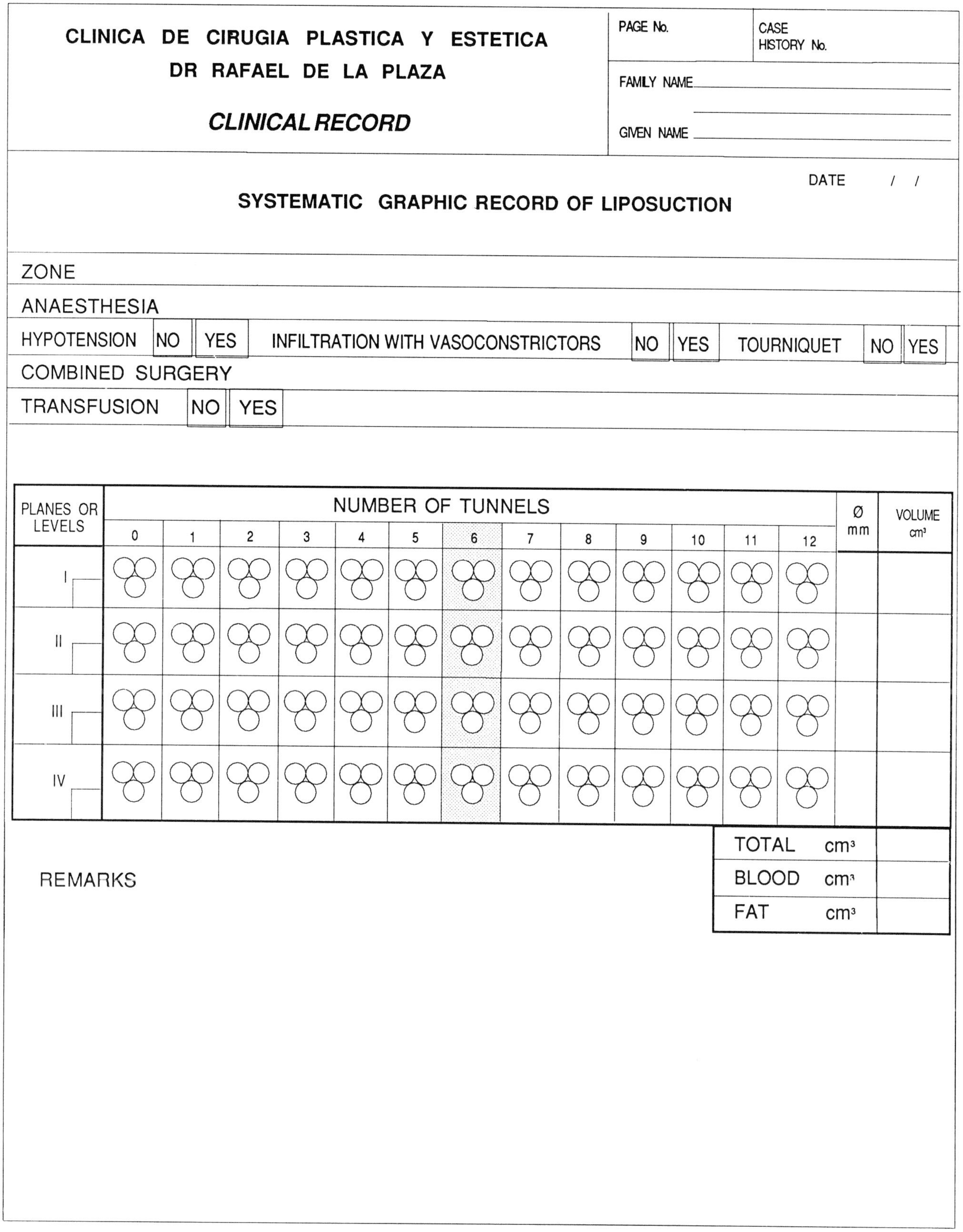

CLINICA DE CIRUGIA PLASTICA Y ESTETICA
DR RAFAEL DE LA PLAZA

CLINICAL RECORD

PAGE No.
CASE HISTORY No.
FAMILY NAME
GIVEN NAME

DATE / /

SYSTEMATIC GRAPHIC RECORD OF LIPOSUCTION

ZONE

ANAESTHESIA

HYPOTENSION NO YES INFILTRATION WITH VASOCONSTRICTORS NO YES TOURNIQUET NO YES

COMBINED SURGERY

TRANSFUSION NO YES

PLANES OR LEVELS	NUMBER OF TUNNELS													Ø mm	VOLUME cm³
	0	1	2	3	4	5	6	7	8	9	10	11	12		
I															
II															
III															
IV															

REMARKS

TOTAL	cm³	
BLOOD	cm³	
FAT	cm³	

A

Figure 3–5. A, B: A clinical record is kept to help the surgeon systematize the technique, record the details, and collect data for statistical studies. *(Figure continues)*

Description of the graph and data registration procedure

PLANES OR LEVELS

Numbers I, II III and IV show the different depths or planes in which the cannula acts, and also the entry points.

ENTRY POINTS

Registered in the column PLANES OR LEVELS with the letters A, B, C, etc., corresponding to the following drawings.

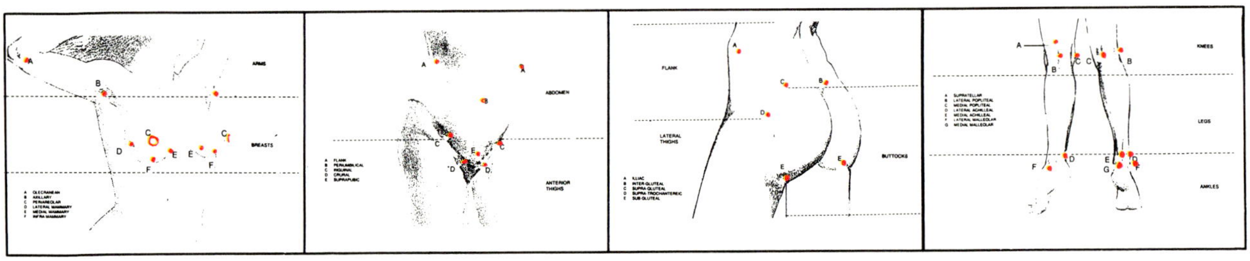

NUMBER OF TUNNELS

Thirteen tunnels are represented (0 to 12) adding tunnels No. 0 and 12 to the Tunnel Tracer. Each tunnel contains a drawing of the three positions that the cannula can take within the tunnel, depending on the position of the aspiration orifices; thus we have three circles: right, left, and lower. In these circles we register the number of strokes made in each of the three positions.

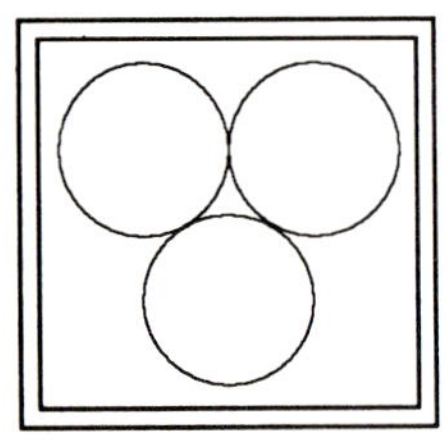

VOLUME cm³

If considered necessary, we register here the volume in cm³ aspirated in each plane or level.

Ø mm

We register the number in mm of the cannula used in each plane or level.

TOTAL cm³	
BLOOD cm³	
FAT cm³	

We add the volumes collected in each plane or level, obtaining the total volume. Blood and fat can be recorded separately if facilities for this are available.

REMARKS

Note will be made of any event occuring during the operation, or additional comments will be made on a specific case as necessary.

In bilateral cases it is not necessary to use two graphs; simply this space for REMARKS will reflect any difference observed with regard to the previously treated side. When there are multiple zones, the last graph will show a final balance of the amounts obtained.

B

Figure 3–5. *(continued)*

arate the concept of what is rational from the purely artistic, since both must be present in every body-contouring surgical procedure. Results using this technique can be seen in Figures 2-2 to 2-4.

INCISIONS

The location and size of the incision in the abdomen will vary according to the classification of the abdomen and the type of surgery. In type I, the only incision is one large enough to introduce the cannulas for SAL. Generally, one incision is placed at the suprapubic area near the hairline and a second in the periumbilical region (Fig. 3-6). We prefer to use two incisions in the flanks, because that allows us to do a crisscross liposuction for a more homogeneous reduction of the fat. These incisions are located in more visible areas, but when using the guided cannulas, skin trauma from friction at the point of penetration is eliminated and a good scar is obtained, which is almost imperceptible. In some cases we can combine a third incision in the periumbilical area if we need to do more suction to rebuild the medial sulcus.

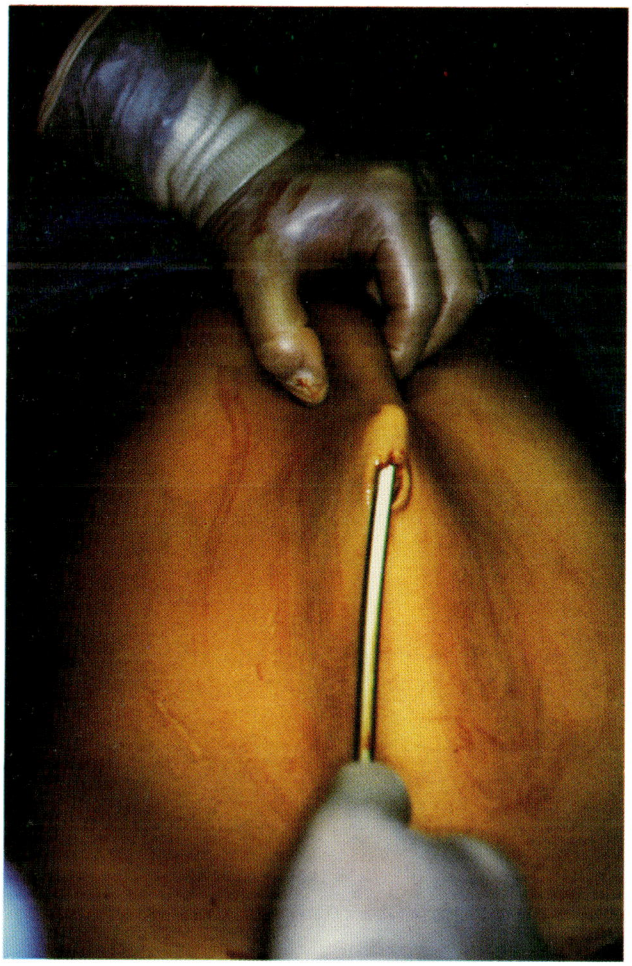

Figure 3-6. Incision inside the navel to facilitate the suction-assisted lipectomy to rebuild the sulcus of the upper abdomen in types I and II.

In types II and III abdomens, a small incision is made, not more than 12 cm in length, immediately over the pubis using one of the creases above the hairline. The closer to the hairline the incision, the less visible it will be in the postoperative period (Fig. 3-7A-C).

In the type IV abdomen, a 20 cm transverse incision is made immediately over the pubis using one of the creases of the skin to allow the undermining of the abdomen in an upward direction to the costal ribs. During surgery, the incision can be increased 5 cm to allow a better view of the upper abdomen with or without detaching the navel (Fig. 3-8A, B).

In the type V abdomen, a 20 to 25 cm transverse incision is made in the inferior abdomen immediately over the pubis, extending inferiorly to the level of the anterior spine of the iliac crest (Fig. 3-9A, B). If the patient has an excess of skin in the hips, the incision may continue more laterally in a variable length up to the posterior axillary line to resect the excess of skin and fat in this region. The incision is transversal and slightly convex over the pubis and concave on the inguinal crease following the natural curvature.

The design of the incision is very important because it will give a scar that will be part of the final aesthetic result of the abdomen. It is important to avoid a high curved incision at the level of the pubis because the scar can work like a "trap door," resulting in a protruded pubis. Other types of incision, such as "W," gull wing, and square incisions, can be used in specific cases, where the goal is to increase the amount of skin resection, but in our opinion it must be avoided because the final scar will not be coincident with the natural creases of the abdomen. In a type VI abdomen, the incision is done in the mammary sulcus from the middle axillary line from one side to the other (Fig. 3-9C).

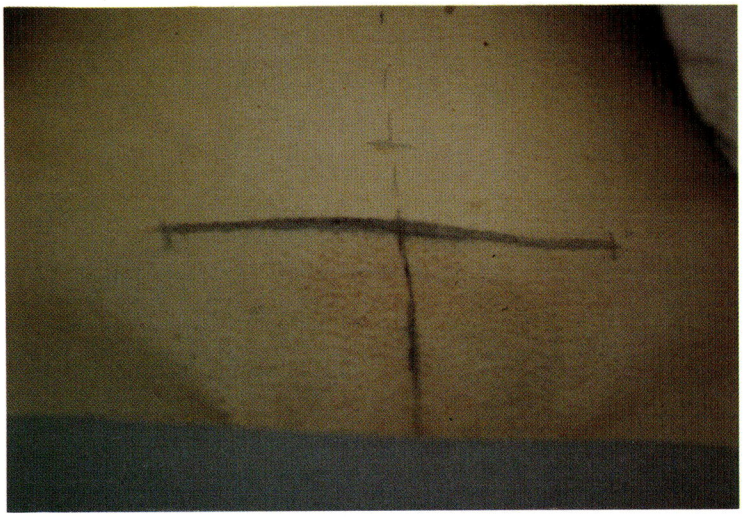

A

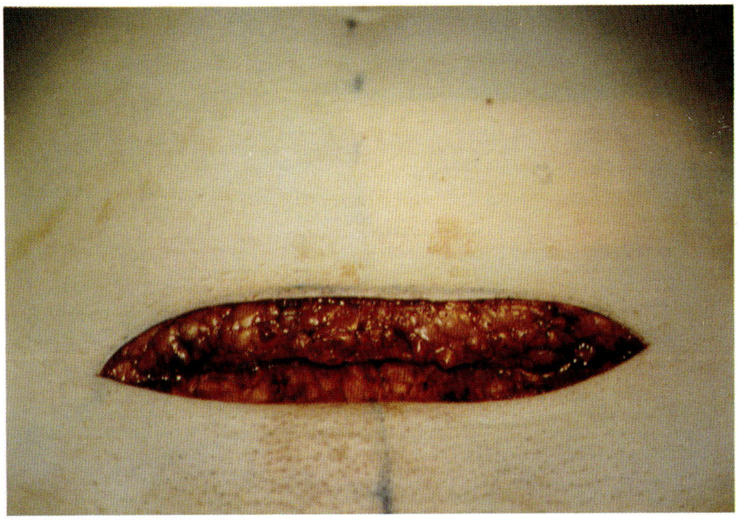

B

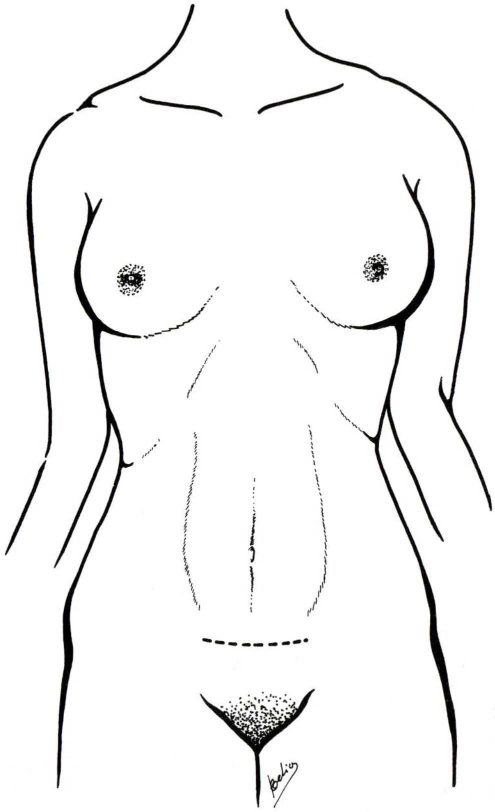

C

Figure 3-7. A-C: Types II and III: incision is 12 cm in length.

DISSECTIONS

The extension of the dissection of the skin from the aponeurotic tissue layer will be variable according to the classification of the abdomen. In the type I abdomen, the only dissection will be made by the cannulas during the liposuction technique. In types II and III the dissection extends from the pubis to the umbilicus and laterally at the anterior axillary line on both sides 5 to 8 cm above the level of the navel. It is important that the cutaneous tissue be completely undermined to allow the reshaping of this skin over the new form of the musculoaponeurotic layer after suturing (Fig. 3-10A, B). In types IV and V, the dissection must be made from the pubis to the margins of the inferior ribs and to the xiphoid (Fig. 3-11). The dissection must reach laterally the anterior axillary line on both sides and continue in an upward direction to the xiphoid in a trapezoidal shape. In the upper abdomen and near the thoracic cage, the dissection is more limited to avoid damage to the perforators of the epigastric vessels, which are situated at the lateral margin of the rectus muscles.

A

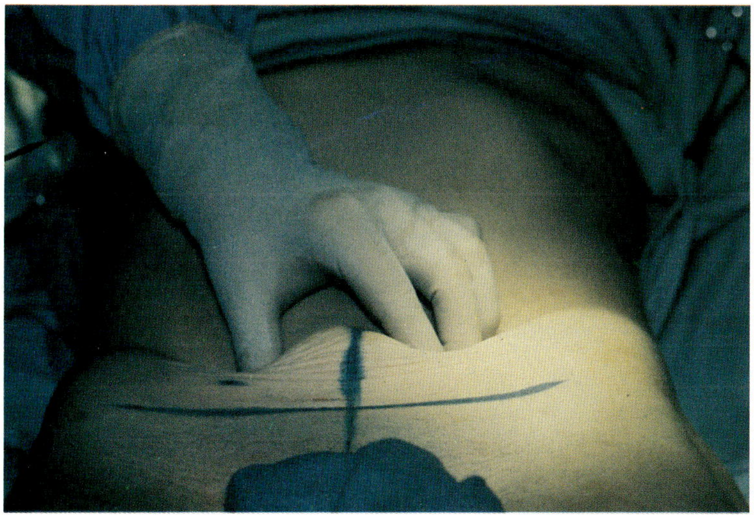

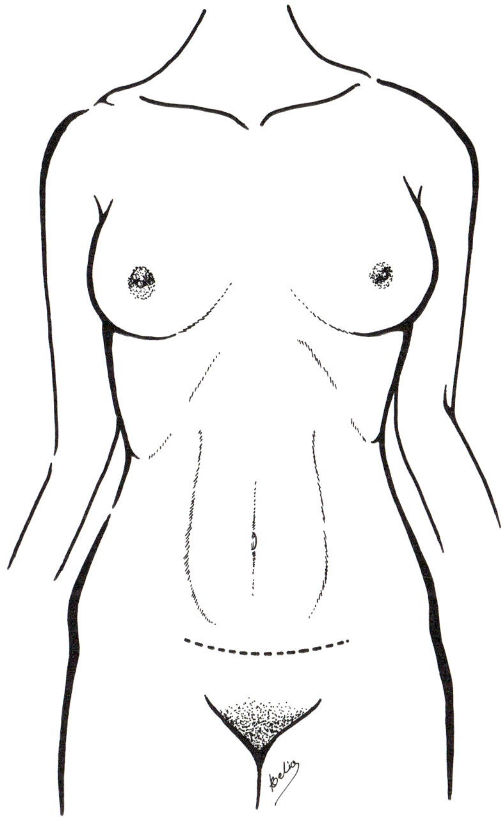

B

Figure 3–8. **A, B:** Type IV: incision is 15 to 20 cm in length along one of the creases of the skin.

A

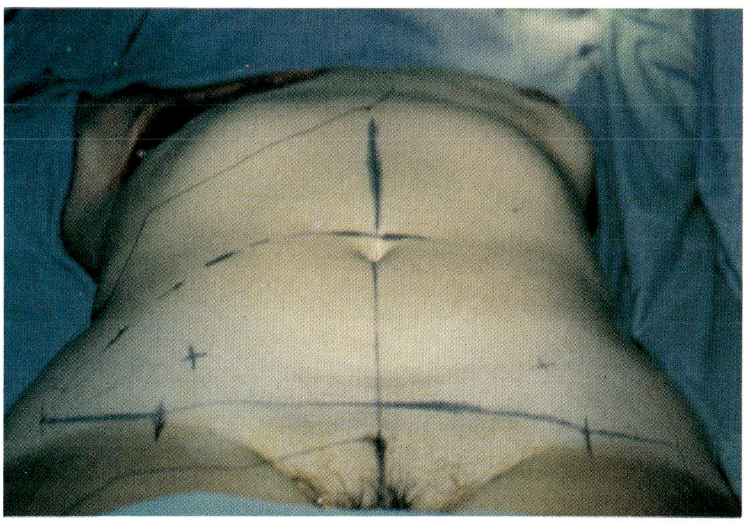

Figure 3–9. **A, B:** Type V: incision with 20 to 25 cm. **C:** Type VI: Schematic drawing of the position of the incision in the mammary sulcus from the middle axillary line on one side to the other. *(Figure continues)*

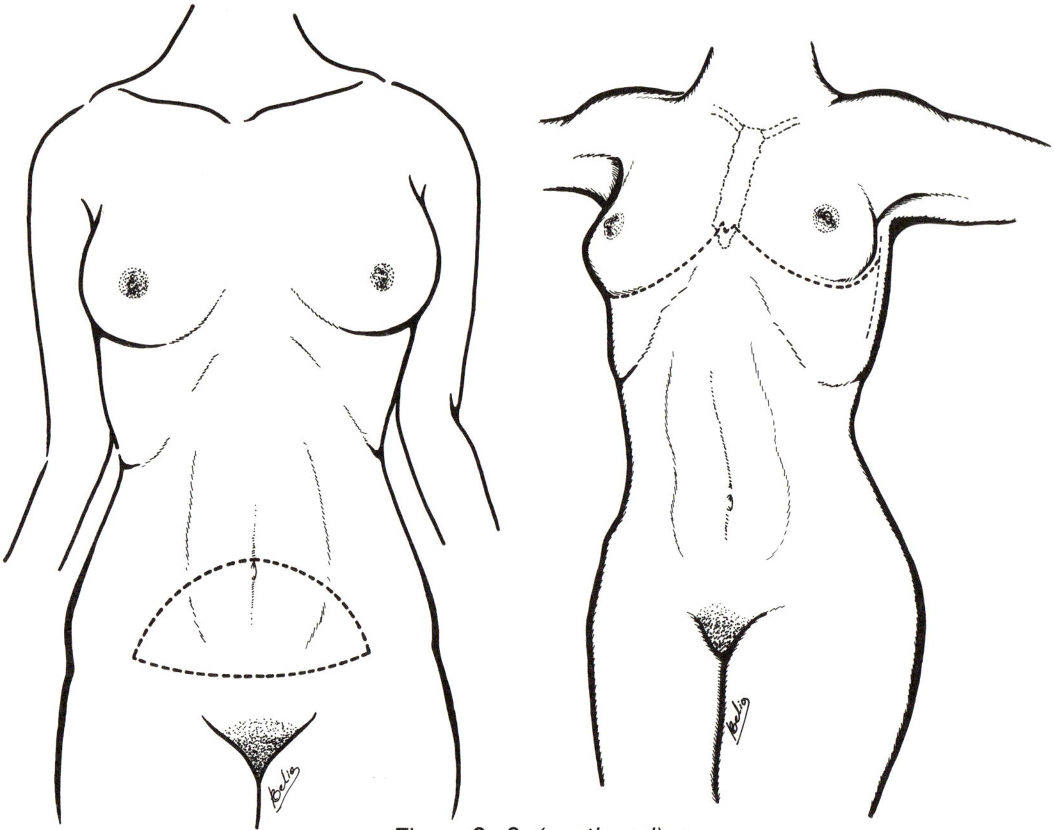

B C

Figure 3–9. *(continued)*

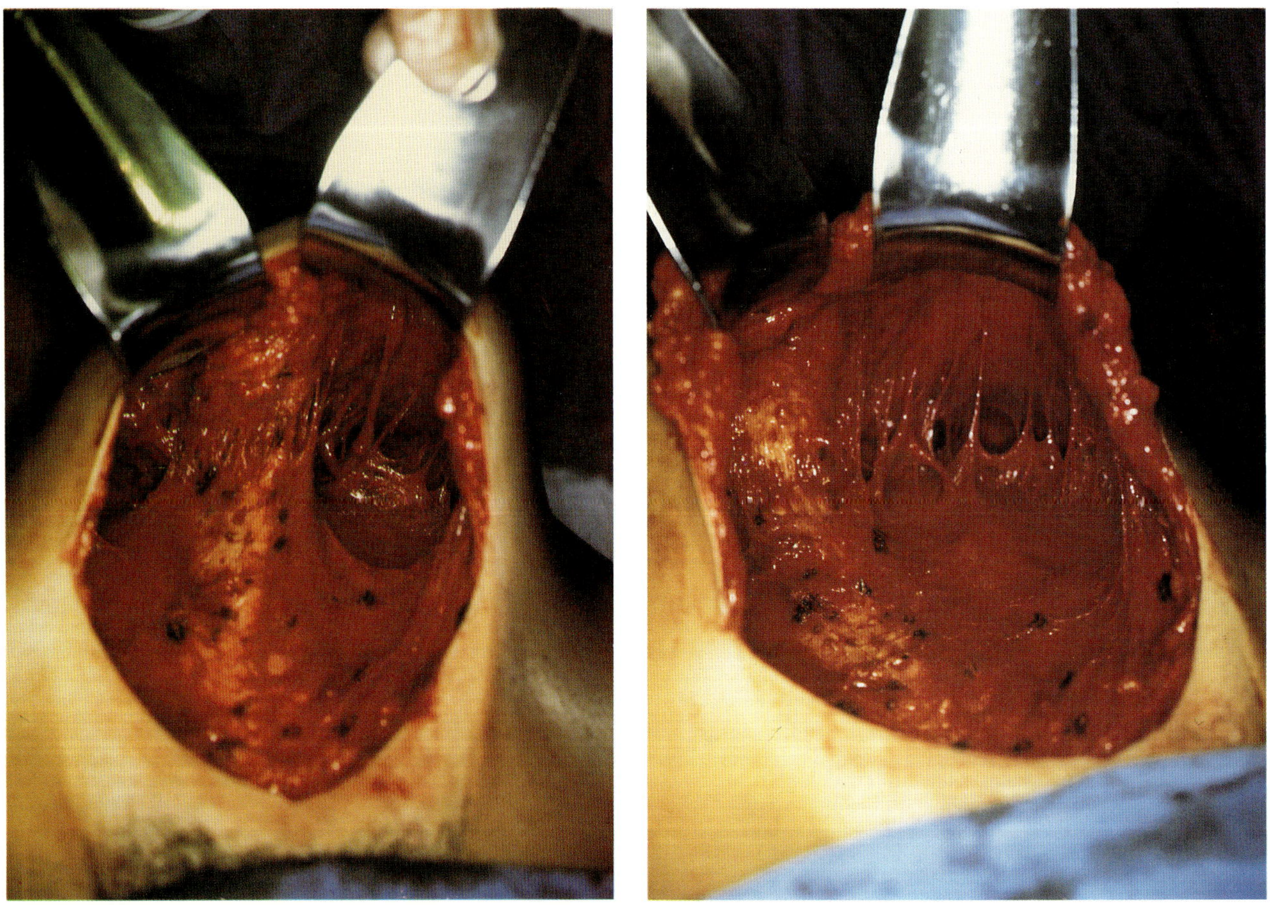

A B

Figure 3–10. A, B: Types II and III: dissection of the cutaneous flap from the pubis to the umbilicus and laterally on both sides 5 to 8 cm above the level of the navel.

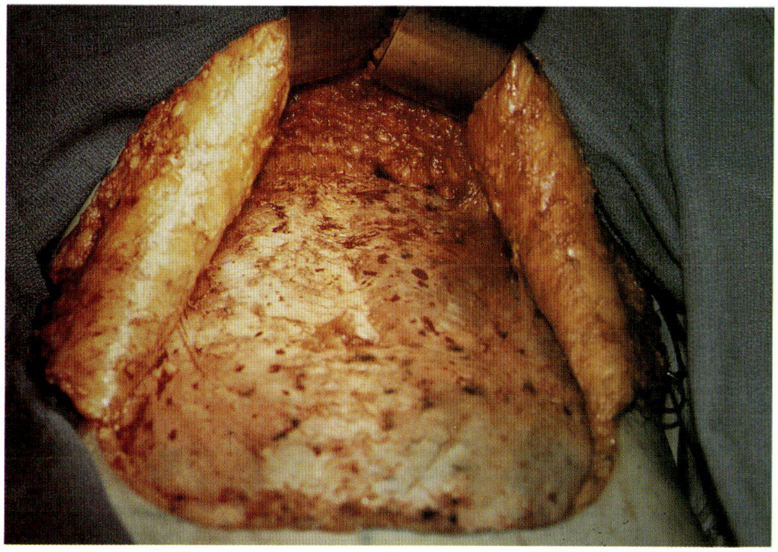

Figure 3–11. Types IV and V: dissection of the cutaneous flap reaches the margin of the inferior ribs and xiphoid.

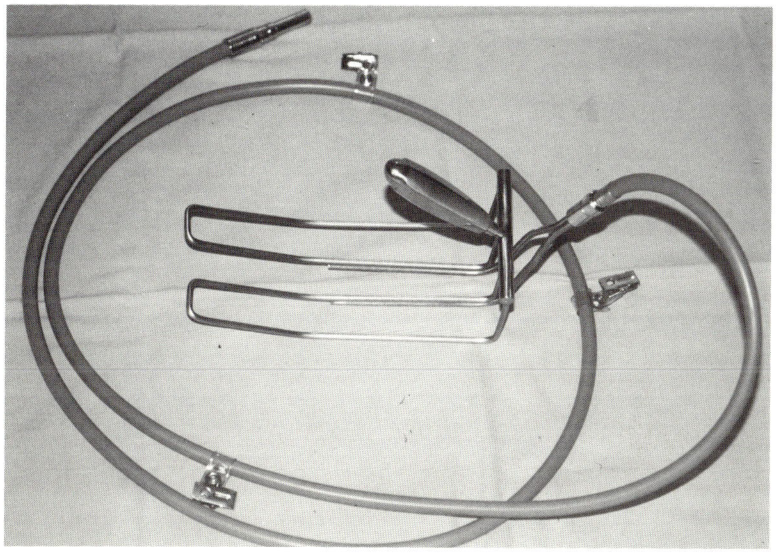

Figure 3–12. Double fiberoptic retractor to facilitate the dissection of the upper abdomen, especially on a type IV abdomen.

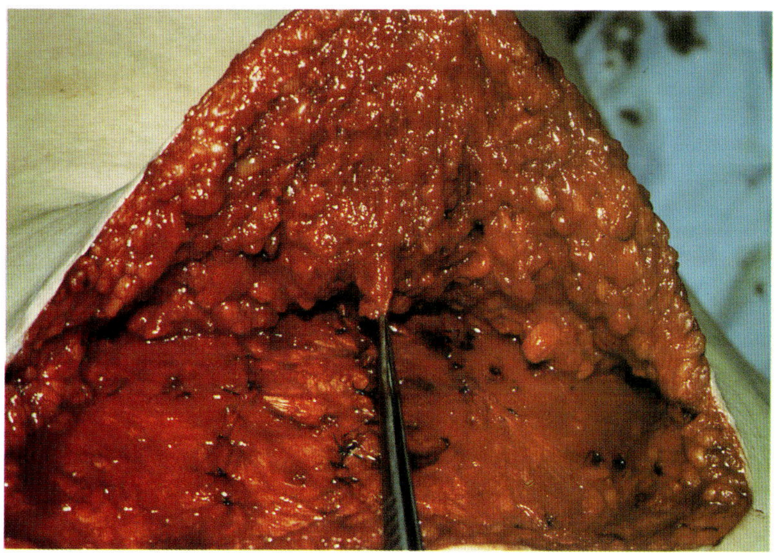

Figure 3–13. Type IV: the navel may be released to dissect the upper part of the abdomen.

In type IV, because there is a smaller incision, it is more difficult to reach the xiphoid. The use of a double fiberoptic retractor facilitates this maneuver (Fig. 3–12). The navel may (Fig. 3–13) or may not be released (Fig. 3–14A, B) in order to reach the upper abdomen better. To allow a good exposure of the upper abdomen, the navel needs to be widely dissected from the subcutaneous tissue and from the aponeurotic layer.

In a type V abdomen, to facilitate the dissection of the upper part of the abdomen, a medial incision is made up to the navel, dividing the abdominal flap (Fig. 3–15).

In type VI, the dissection is extended to the level of the navel and laterally downward to this level (Fig. 3–16).

MUSCULAR APONEUROTIC ALTERATIONS

The abdomen is a complex structure. The external and internal oblique and transverse abdominal muscles are situated laterally, and the rectus muscles and aponeurosis, medially.

During pregnancy these muscles relax and increase in size due to hormonal action and the growth of the fetus (Fig. 3–17A, B). This augmentation of the musculoaponeurotic layer occurs in all directions in a short period of time. After pregnancy, this phenomenon is reversed to a variable degree, one that is unique to each individual woman, resulting in several gradations of skin excess and musculoaponeurotic laxity. An overall

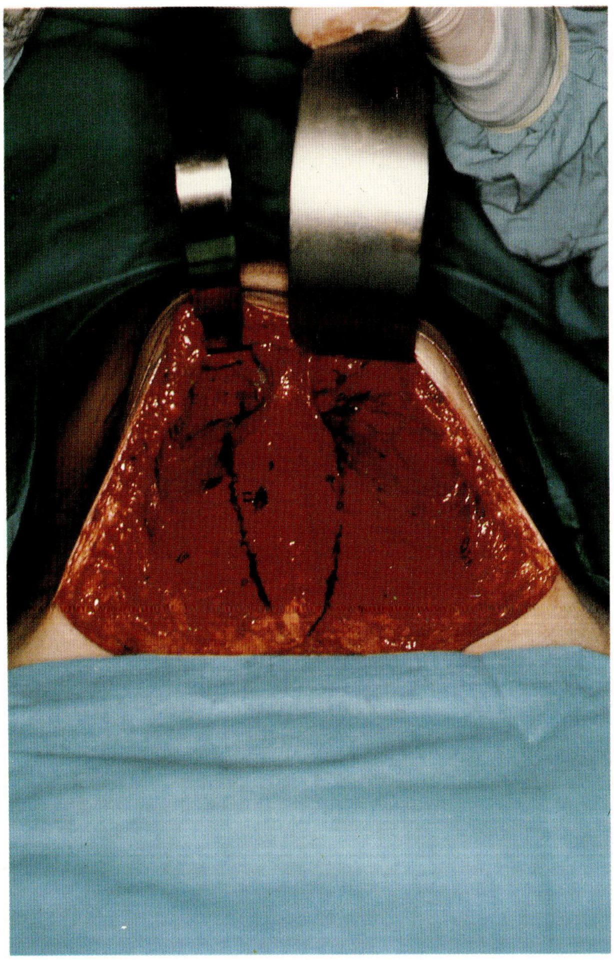

A

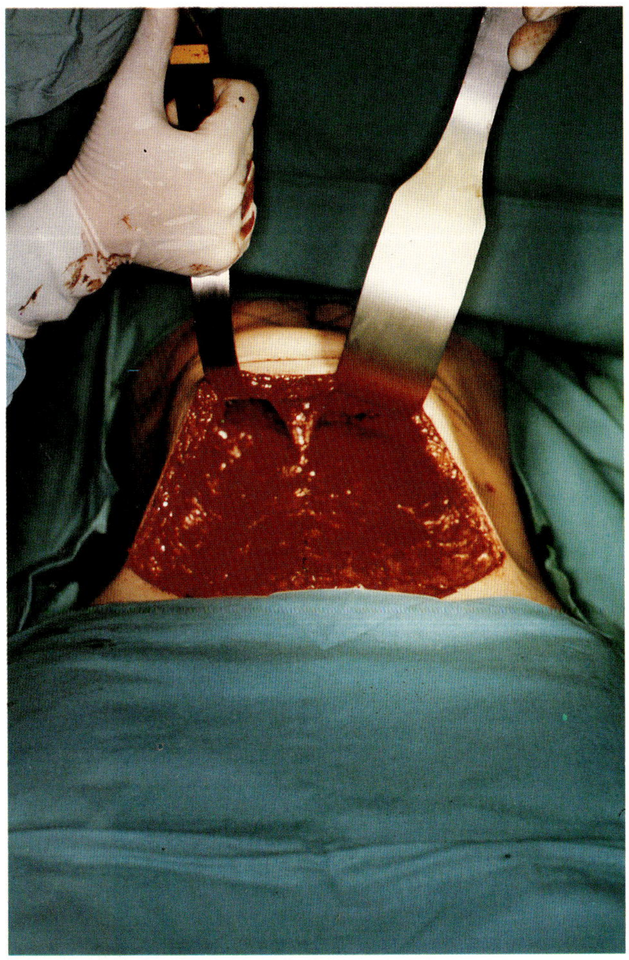

B

Figure 3–14. A: Type IV: to dissect the upper abdomen the navel need not be released. A wide dissection around it exposes the upper abdomen. The margins of the rectus muscles are marked with methylene blue. B: The situation after plicature of the muscles.

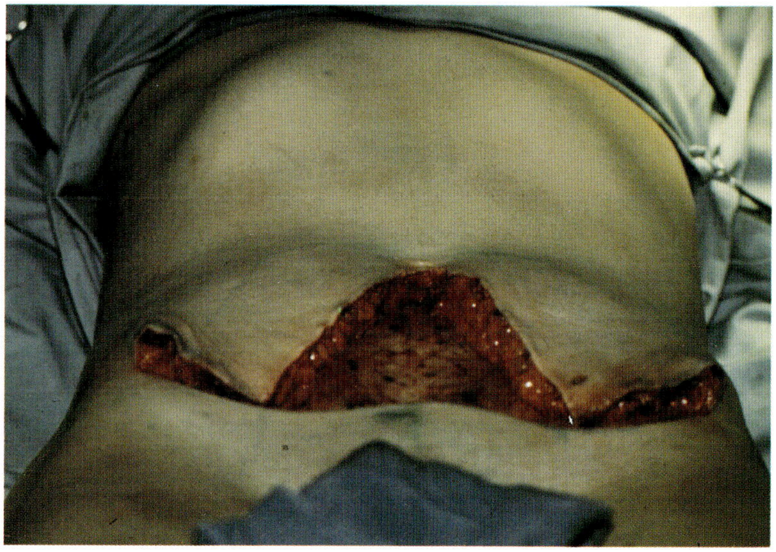

Figure 3–15. Type V: to facilitate the dissection of the upper part of the abdomen, the flap is divided in the midline up to the umbilicus.

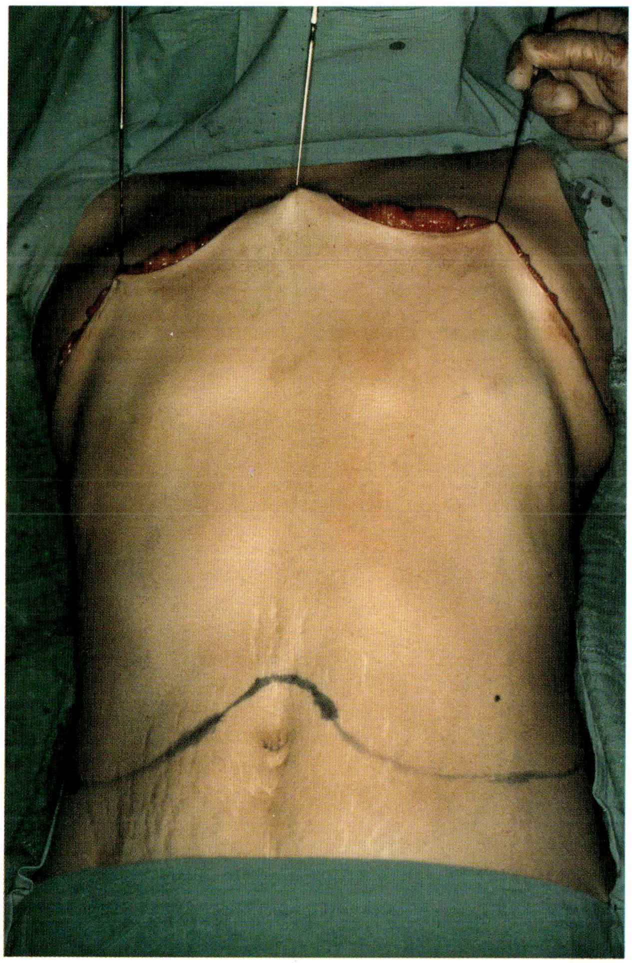

Figure 3–16. In type VI the dissection is performed to the level of the navel and lower laterally, as can be seen by the ink mark.

flaccidity of the abdominal muscles is what is generally found in postpartum patients, and in many of them the distance between the inner margins of the rectus muscles is increased, as well as that between the inner margins of the oblique muscles (diastasis) (Fig. 3–18). The vertical arch formed by the rectus muscles and aponeurosis from the xiphoid to the pubis is also augmented, producing the anterior protuberance of the abdomen (see Fig. 3–20).

RECTUS MUSCLE APONEUROSIS PLICATION

The diastasis of the rectus muscles is not seen in all cases of abdominoplasty. Normally, the distance between them is 2 to 5 cm at their inner margins. We consider a diastasis to have occurred when this distance is greater than normal, even though in many patients in whom the distance is normal, plication is needed to correct the overall flaccidity of the aponeurotic layer as well as to reduce the arch between the xiphoid and the pubis.

The plication is made with sutures of strong nonabsorbable material, preferably with interrupted stitches because they are safer. Also, an interrupted "U" suture can be used (Fig. 3–19). If continuous sutures are used, they must be reinforced with several interrupted stitches to guarantee the continuity of the suture line and avoid reoccur-

A

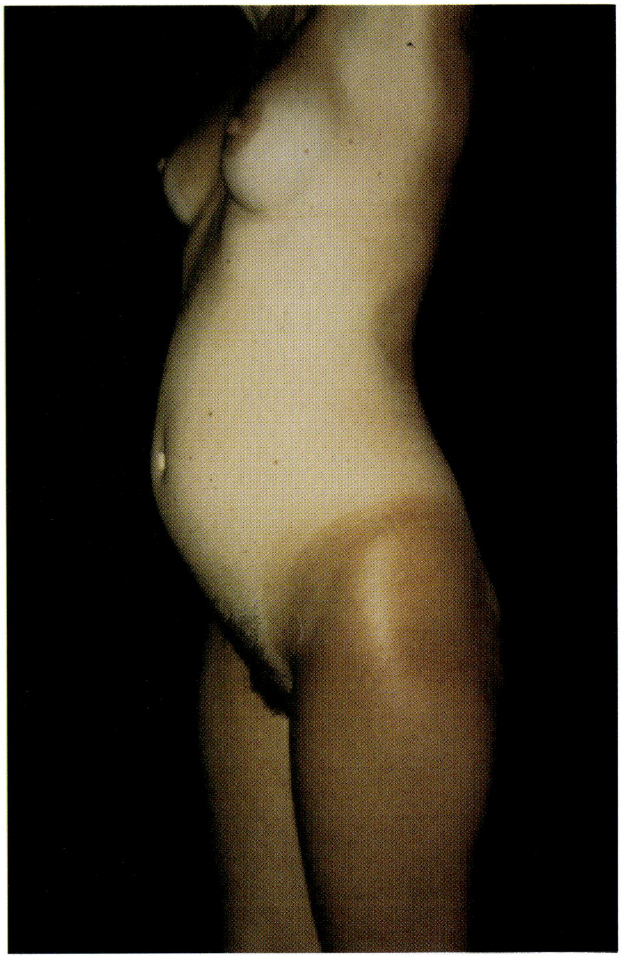

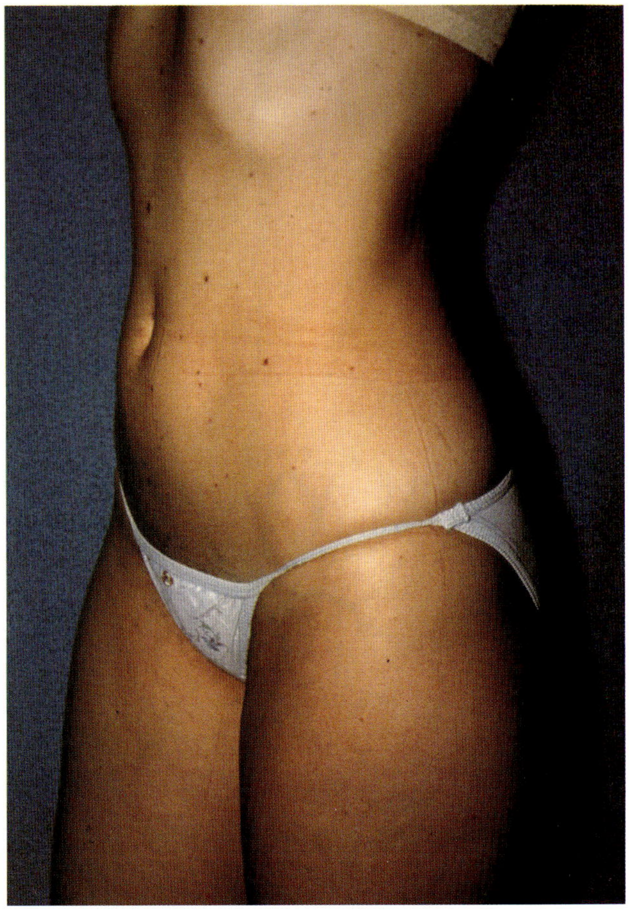

B

Figure 3-17. A, B: Patient during and after pregnancy; the abdominal muscles relax with stretching of the musculoaponeurotic layer and diastasis of the rectus and oblique muscles.

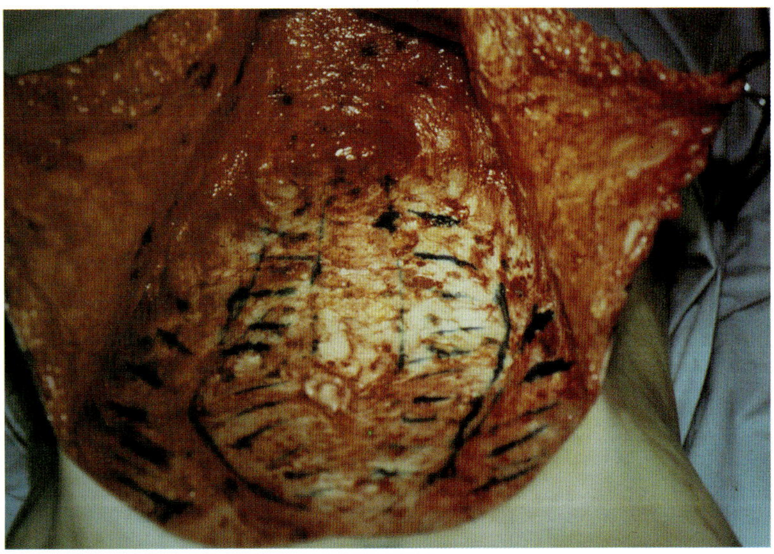

Figure 3-18. Intraoperative aspect of the rectus and oblique muscle diastasis.

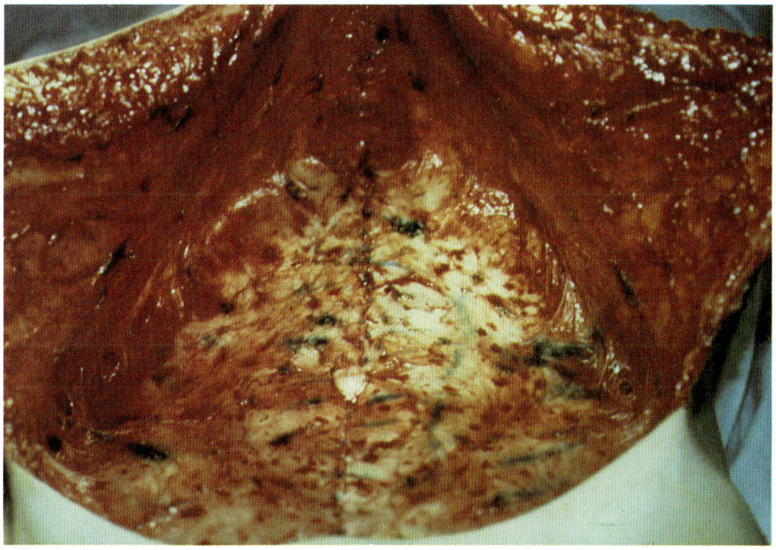

Figure 3–19. The diastasis of the rectus muscles is preferably corrected by suturing with strong nonabsorbable interrupted stitches.

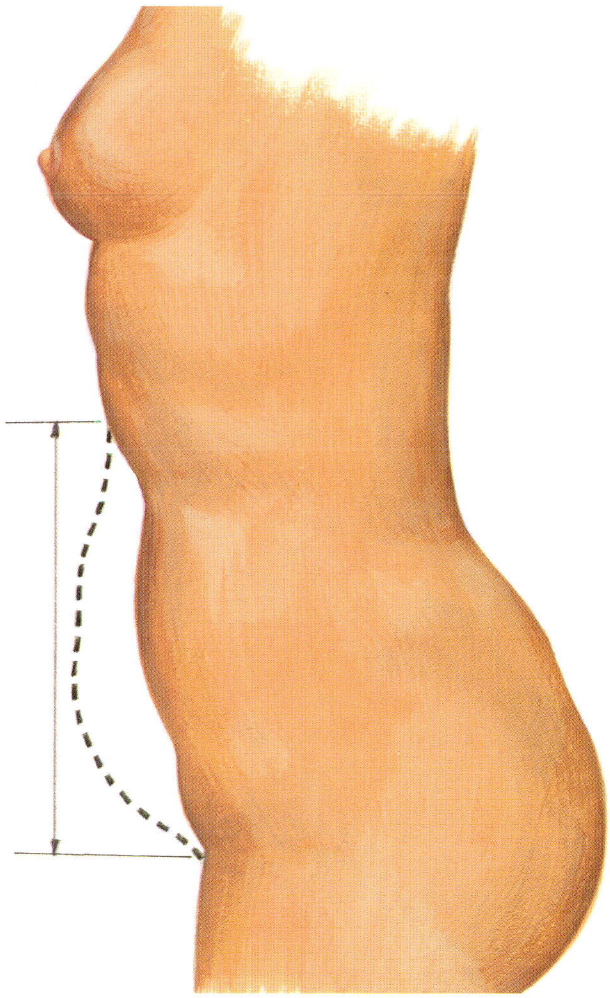

Figure 3–20. The plicature of the rectus muscles to correct the anterior prominence of the abdomen by rectification of the arch between the xiphoid and pubis. (Drawing by S. Sanni.)

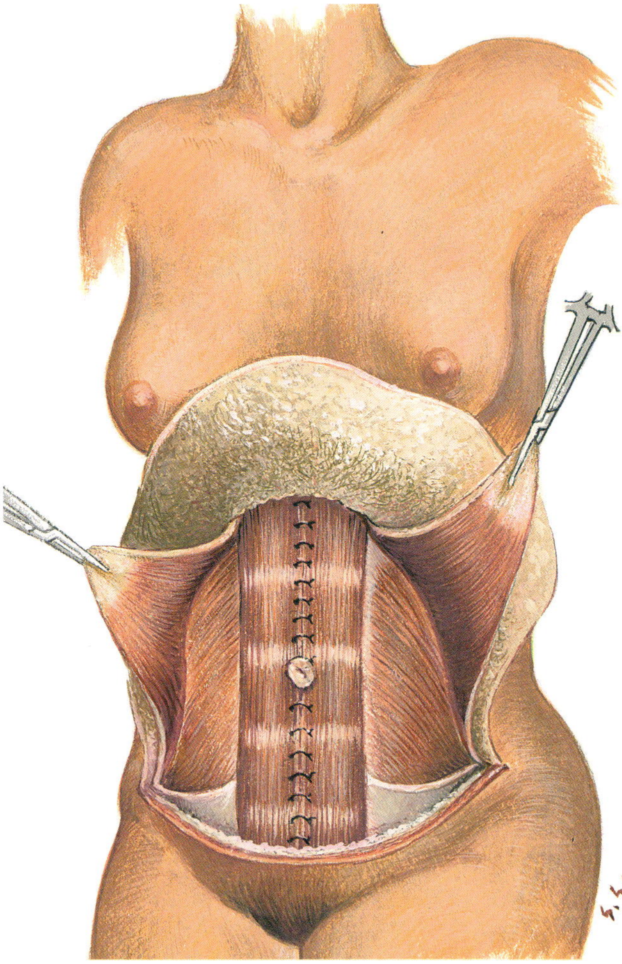

A

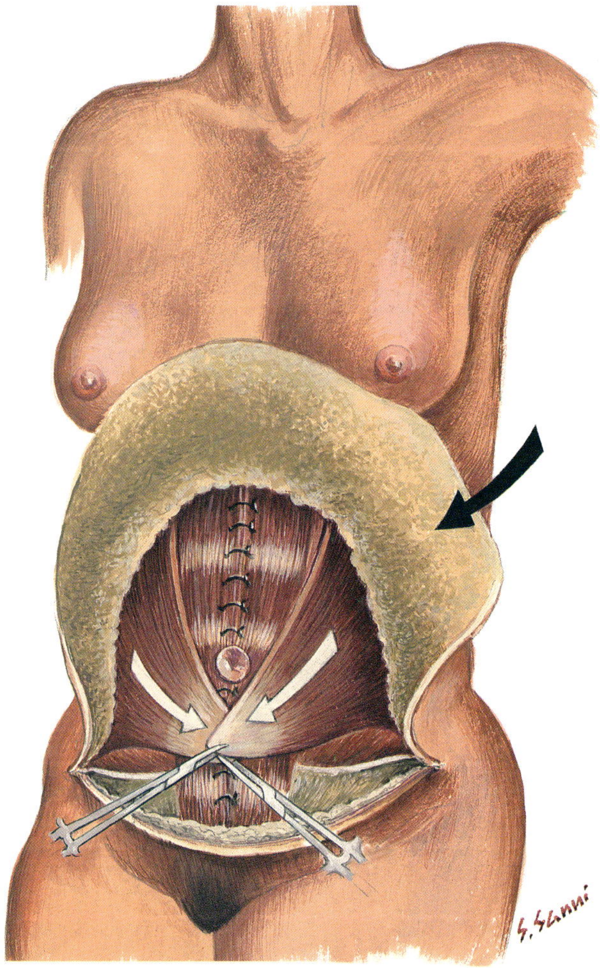

B

Figure 3–21. A–D: Schema of the advancement of the external oblique muscle technique with the goals to reduce the waist, to reshape the semilunar lines, and to reshape the medial depression to the iliac crest.

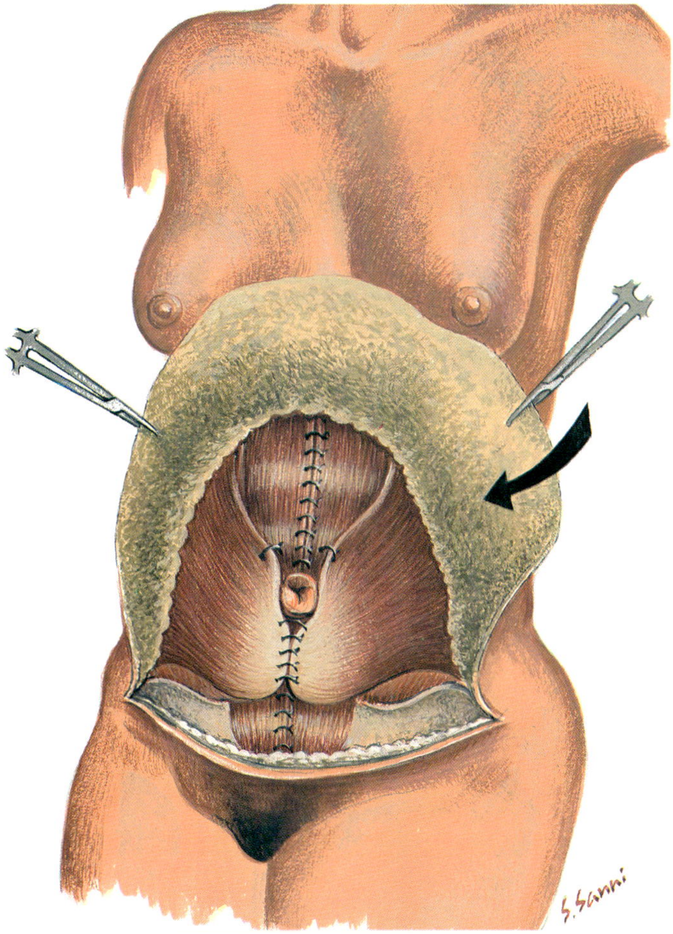

C

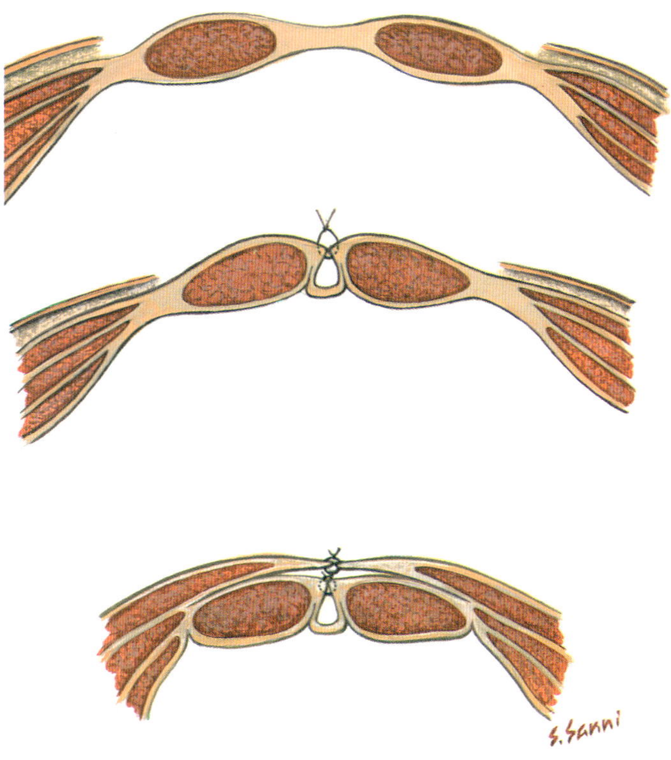

Figure 3-21. *(continued)*

D

rence of the diastasis. The suture is first located from the xiphoid to the navel, and from the umbilicus to the pubis, or vice-versa. This plication reduces the anterior prominence of the abdomen obtained by the rectification of the arch formed by the rectus muscles between the xiphoid and the pubis (Fig. 3–20).

OBLIQUE MUSCLE ADVANCEMENT TECHNIQUE (PSILLAKIS)

Surgical dissection of the external oblique muscle is important to restore the size of the waist, which was enlarged during pregnancy, and to shape the abdomen in a more natural and aesthetic form.

The internal oblique muscle has also been used, but without result because the muscle is very small. The action of the external oblique muscle over the internal and transverse abdominis is enough to obtain a good result.

Several techniques have been tried by us and can be used in different situations. They will be described here. Ours is not the final word on the subject, but the judgment attained through experience of the readers will provide the final answer. However, our experience comes from the treatment of a large number of patients, with very satisfactory results.

The size of the waist, the area between the inferior ribs and the hips, depends on the thickness of the cutaneous tissue and the position of the external and internal oblique and transverse muscles. The plication of the rectus muscles from the xiphoid to the pubis does not alter the waist. To obtain reduction of the waist, the external oblique muscle must be medialized and the fat of the subcutaneous tissue reduced. To medialize the external oblique muscle, dissection and mobilization in a medial and downward direction is better than simple plication, which we have used for many years. Its action over the internal and transverse muscle will be enough to give a good contour to the waist with a simple minor procedure (Fig. 3–21A–D).

To dissect the external oblique muscle, a small incision is made in the lateral margin of the rectus muscles in the inferior abdomen to find the space between the aponeurosis of the external and internal oblique muscles (Fig. 3–22). With scissors or with the finger, we can easily find the avascular plane that exists between them (Fig. 3–23). The inner margin of the external oblique aponeurosis is separated from the lateral margin of the rectus muscles (Fig. 3–24A–D). The aponeurosis of the external oblique muscle must be opened from the most inferior extremity at the suprapubic area up to the ribs, in a curved shape with its convex side directed to the midline. Laterally, the dissection of the oblique muscle must extend to the anterior axillary line where there are several pedicles (Fig.

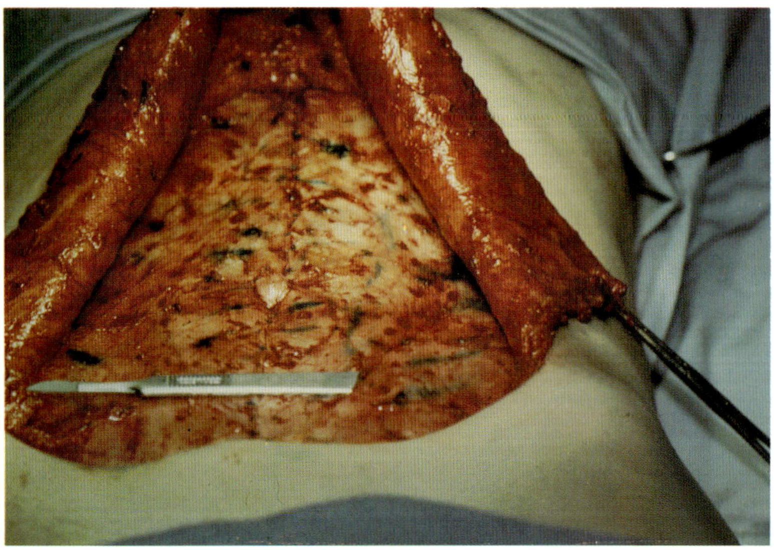

Figure 3–22. Intraoperative view of the external oblique muscle advancement technique: the dissection of the external oblique muscles begins with a small incision in the inferior part of the abdomen lateral to the external margin of the rectus muscle. We can see the handle of the knife under the aponeurosis of the external oblique muscle.

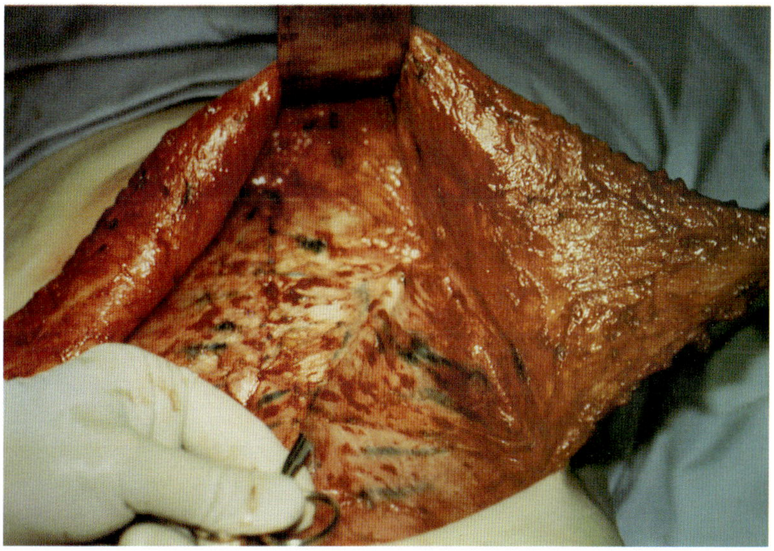

Figure 3–23. With scissors or with the finger, the avascular plane between the external and internal oblique muscles is easily found. We can see the scissors under the external oblique muscle near the margin of the rectus abdominis muscle.

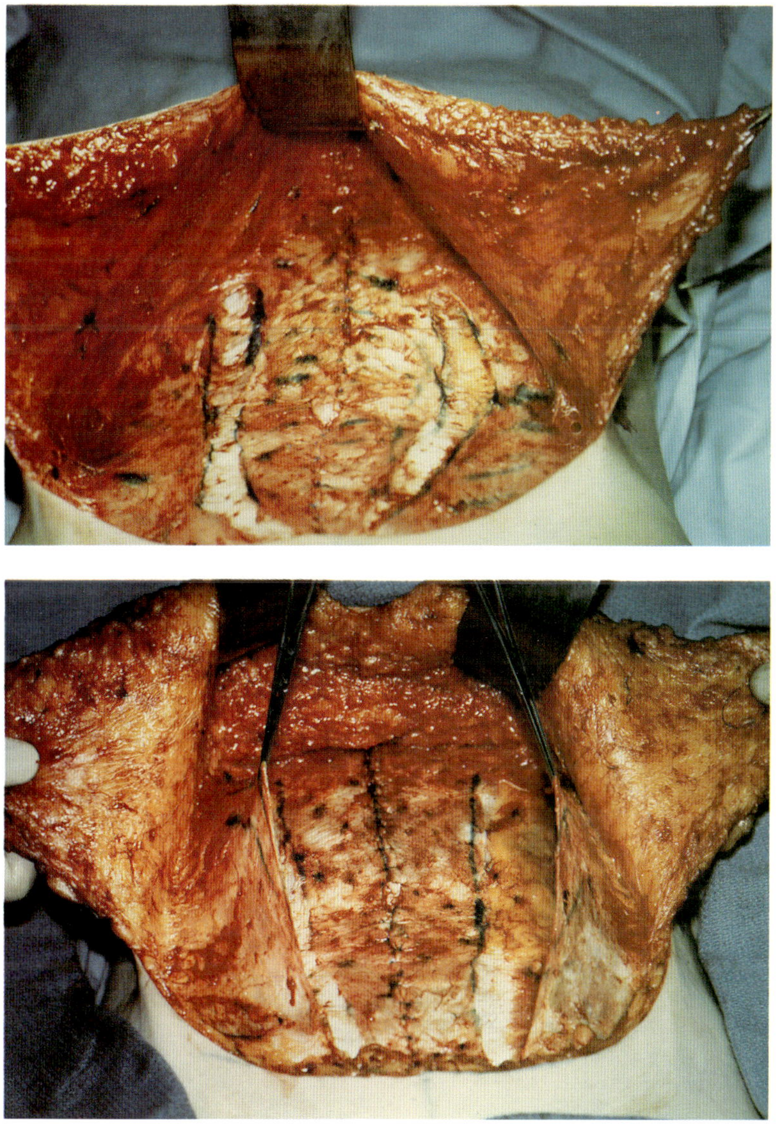

A

B

Figure 3–24. A, B: The inner margins of the external oblique muscles are separated from the lateral margin of the rectus muscles.

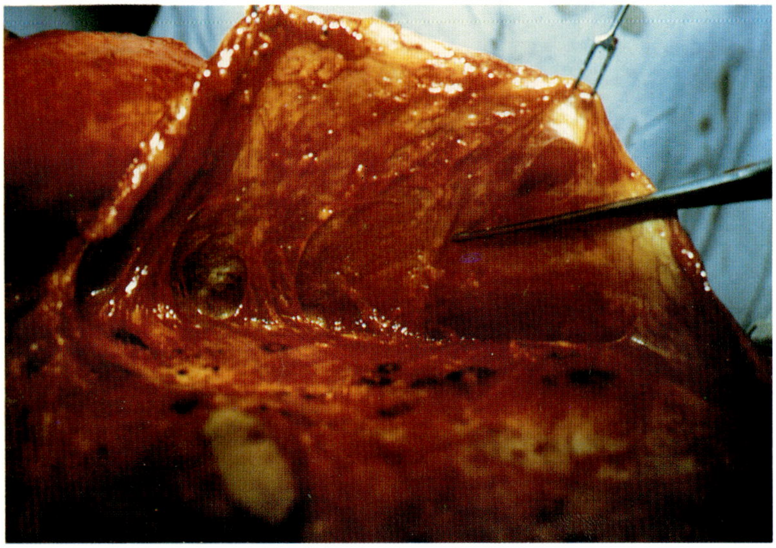

Figure 3–25. Several pedicles of the external oblique muscle.

A

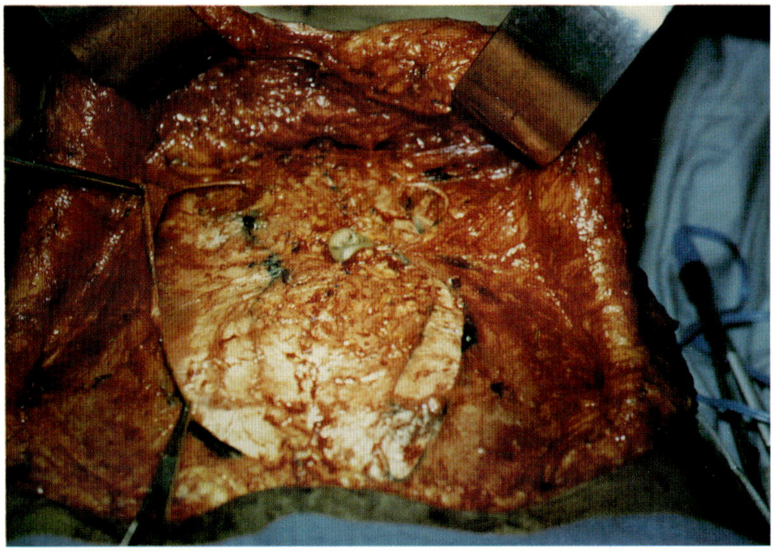

B

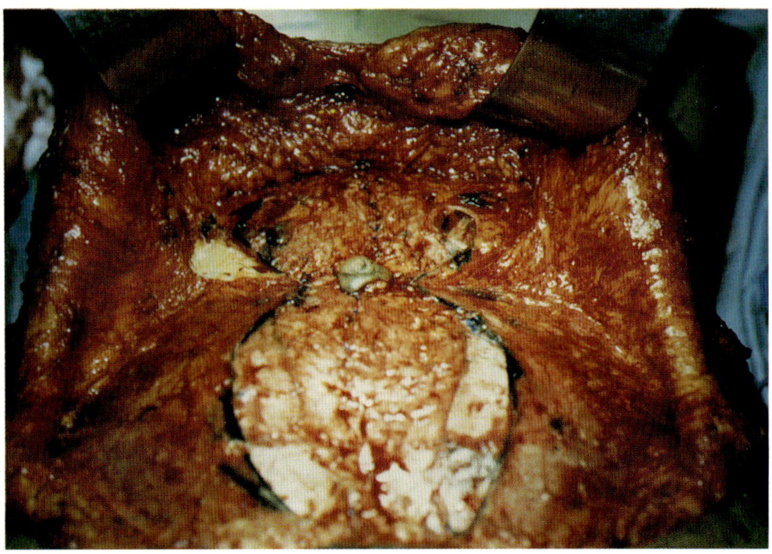

Figure 3–26. A, B: The first two stitches are placed bilaterally at the level of the navel to avoid distortion of the position of the navel from the midline.

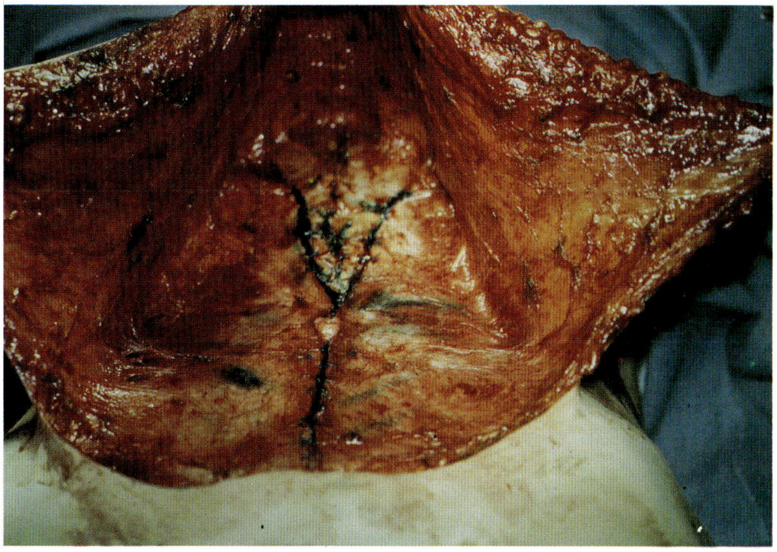

A

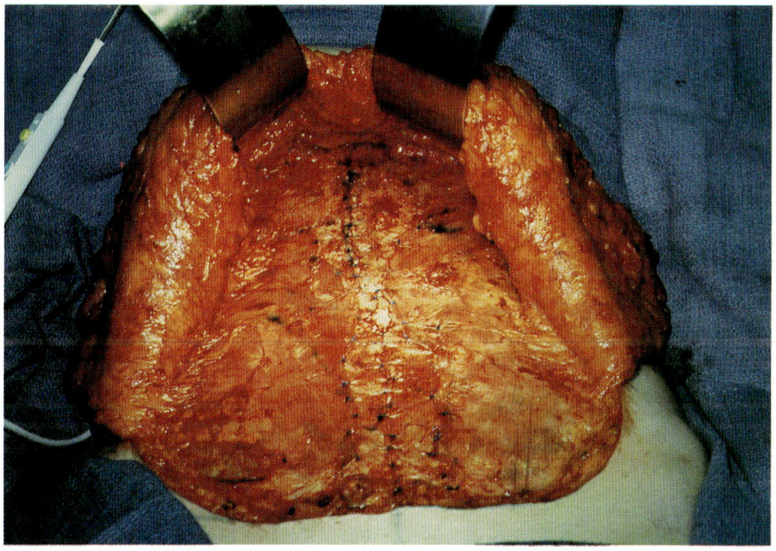

B

Figure 3–27. A, B: The external oblique muscles are sutured with interrupted nonabsorbed stitches along all of the margins. Two examples of the final position of the muscles.

3–25). Care must be taken to avoid damage to them. After the dissection, the muscle is pulled in a downward and medial direction to reduce the waist. Sometimes the flaccidity is so severe that the muscle will extend beyond the midline. The first two sutures must be placed at the level of the navel on both sides to avoid distortion of its position from the midline (Fig. 3–26A, B). Sutures are completed with interrupted stitches with nonabsorbable material (Fig. 3–27A, B). The reduction of the waist by this method can be seen in Table 3–1 depicting the measurements of a series of 20 patients .

SUPERIMPOSITION OF THE EXTERNAL OBLIQUE MUSCLE (APPIANI)

The external oblique muscle is divided by an incision from the pubic region to the midaxillary line at the level of the inferior ribs between the 10th and the 11th perforating rami of the intercostal nerves to avoid damage to the pedicle (Fig. 3–28A–C). The separation of the muscle should be made with scissors following the direction of the muscle fibers. The muscle flaps are separated from the internal oblique muscles and the exter-

Table 3-1. Pre- and Postoperative Measurements of the Waist in 20 Patients with External Oblique Muscle Surgery

		WEIGHT (kg)		WAIST (cm)	
PATIENT	*AGE*	*Preoperative*	*Postoperative*	*Preoperative*	*Postoperative*
1	45	58	58	80	78
2	38	69	73	92	82
3	44	54	53	78	73
4	36	52	57	80	80
5	28	73	66	101	80
6	25	69	63	85	78
7	36	71	64	96	80
8	48	62	63	80	73
9	43	68	66	90	83
10	40	53	51	77	73
11	51	63	64	86	85
12	55	66	63	83	76
13	47	61	55	81	76
14	44	56	56	75	71
15	48	60	59	92	81
16	36	65	69	81	78
17	50	57	55	91	77
18	37	57	57	75	73
19	26	56	58	87	75
20	36	56	52	75	73

nal flap is widely dissected to facilitate the superimposition of the flaps. The internal flap is sutured laterally by transfixing stitches to the external one in an arch line. To reinforce the previous suture, a second layer of stitches is placed parallel to the first. The margin of the external flap is fixed by a continuous suture. The position of this suture is variable, according to the laxity of the muscles, and in the most flaccid cases the flaps can be superimposed on the fascia of the rectus sheath.

GIRDLE MUSCLE FLAP PROCEDURE (APPIANI)

Type I

This procedure is employed in patients with minor relaxation of the musculoaponeurotic layer. On the external oblique muscle, a flap 5 to 7 cm wide is drawn in the direction of the muscle fibers, including the 10th and 11th posterior perforating rami of the intercostal nerves (Fig. 3-29A-C). Using knife and scissors, the flap of the external oblique muscle is lifted. The upper end of the pedicle should reach the costal margin. The edges of the donor side of the external oblique muscle are sutured by interrupted stitches, which will produce muscle continuity and modeling of the waist. Both muscle flaps are carried toward the anterior medial line below the umbilicus, where they are crossed, superimposed, and sutured to each other.

Type II

When there are cases with great laxity of the musculoaponeurotic layer in a protruded abdomen, it is necessary to conduct the following procedure. At the level of the flank, a fold of the major oblique muscle is pinched in an effort to achieve the largest fold possible. Two flaps 6 to 9 cm in width are drawn downward, including the lateral branches of the 10th and 11th intercostal nerves, and passing below the navel. The incision in the muscle is made parallel to its fibers in the direc-

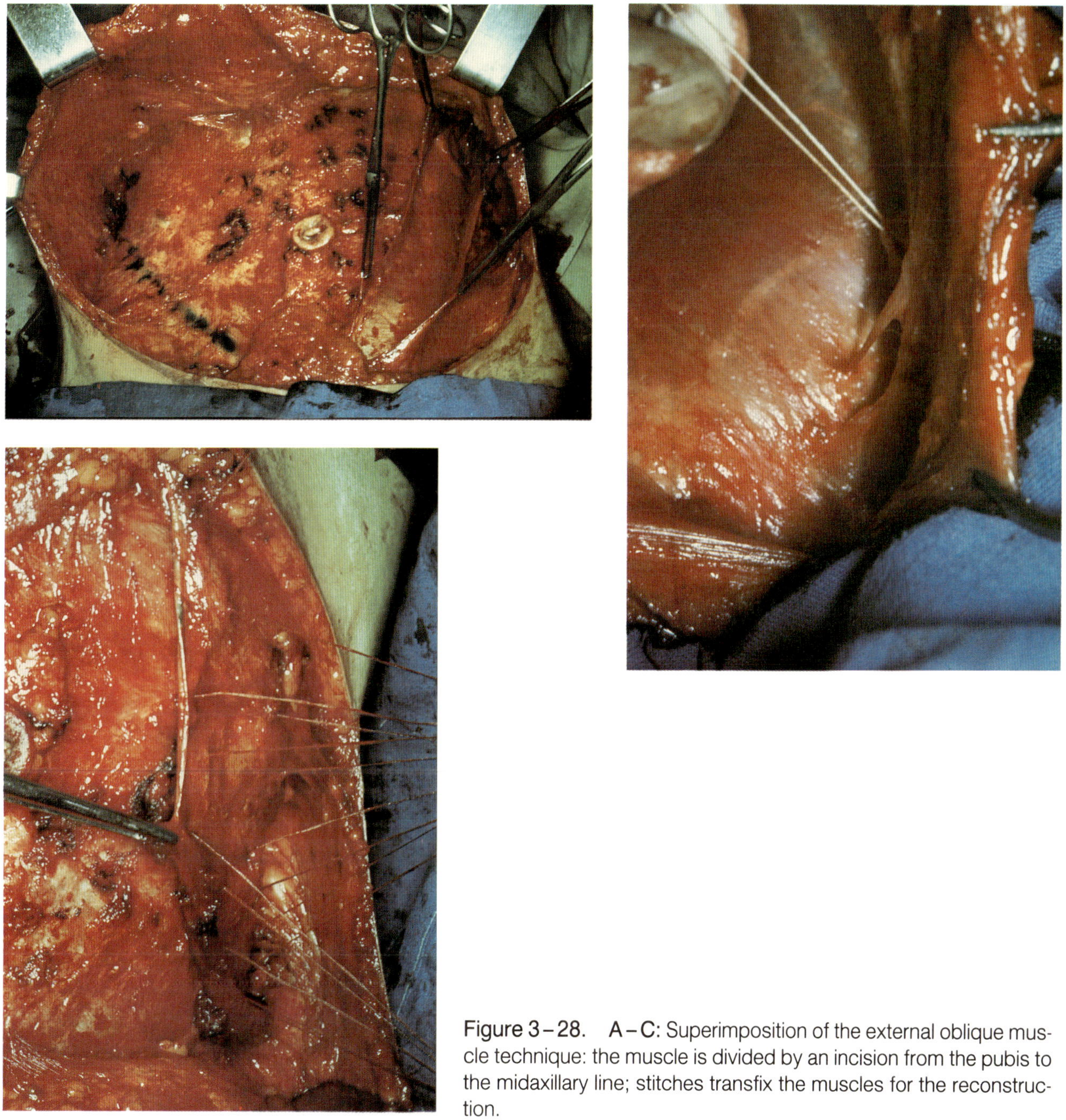

A

B

C

Figure 3-28. A-C: Superimposition of the external oblique muscle technique: the muscle is divided by an incision from the pubis to the midaxillary line; stitches transfix the muscles for the reconstruction.

tion of the exterior border of the rectus muscle, and the anterior sheath is included as a unit (Fig. 3-30A-D).

If there is no rectus diastasis to simplify the technique, the flap can be elevated as a unit and then divided in the midline (Fig. 3-31).

The borders of the donor area are brought together with separate stitches in the external oblique muscle and the recti abdominis sheath, restoring the anatomic unity. Both musculoaponeurotic flaps are lifted forward in order to cross in the waist like a belt.

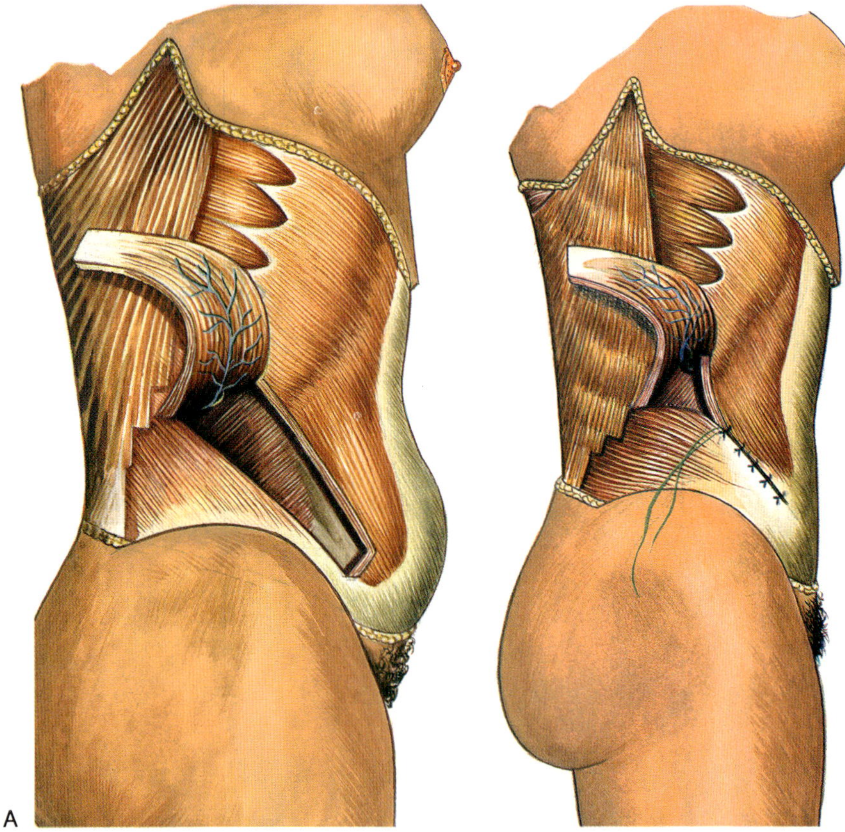

A B

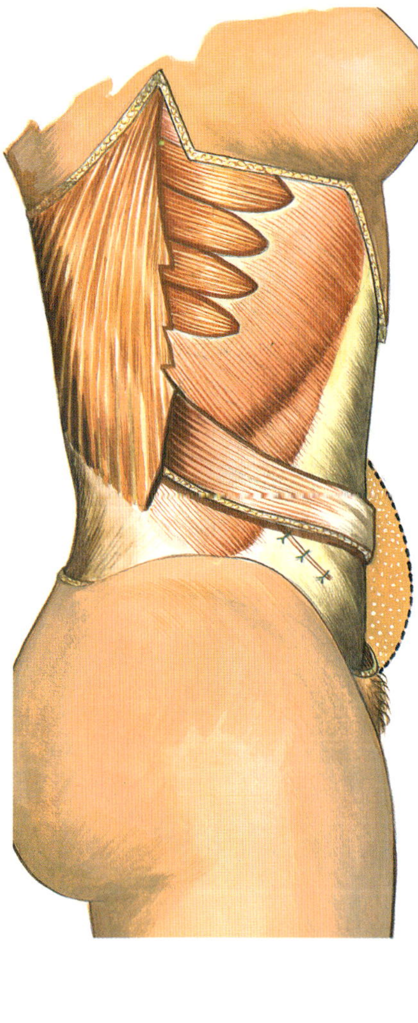

C

Figure 3–29. A–C: Schematic drawings of the girdle muscle procedure to reduce the waist. (Drawings by Franz W. Guzmán.)

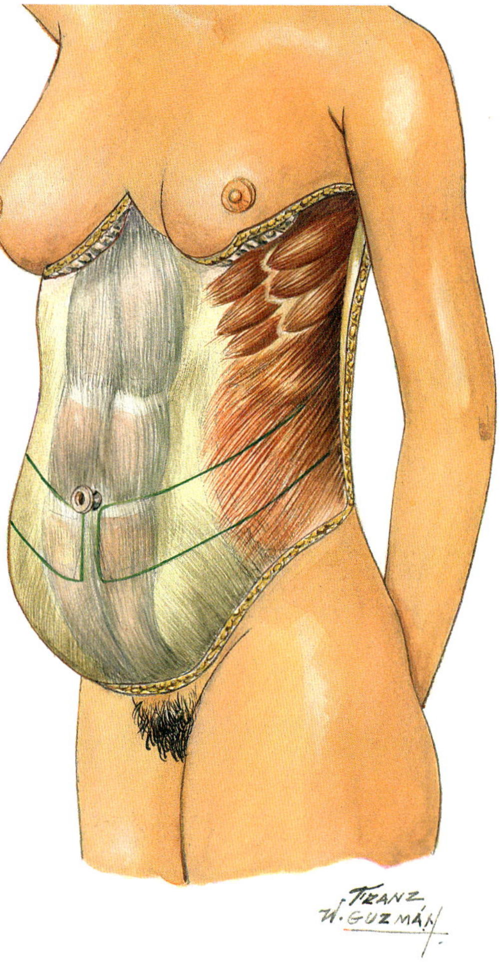

A

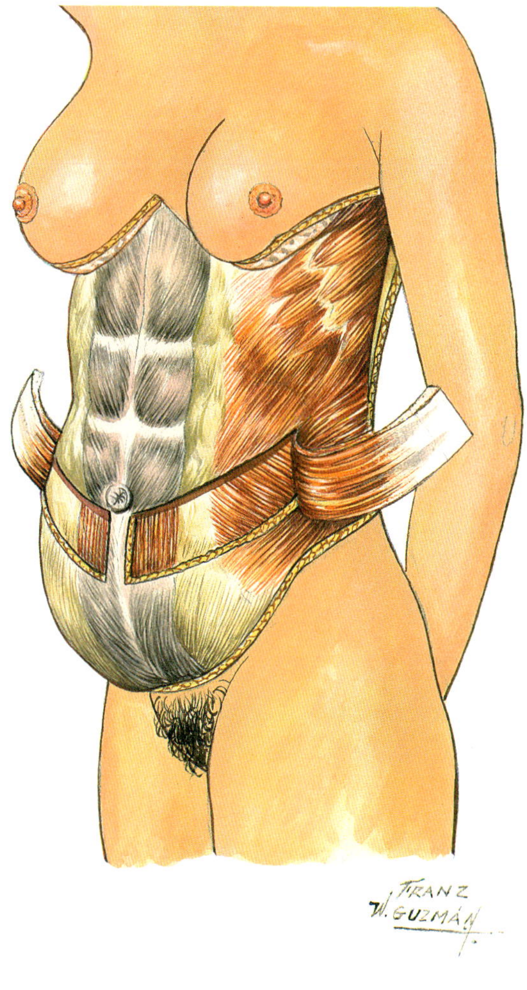

B

Figure 3–30. A–D: Schematic drawings of the girdle muscle procedure in cases of great laxity of the abdominal aponeurotic layer. *(Figure continues)*

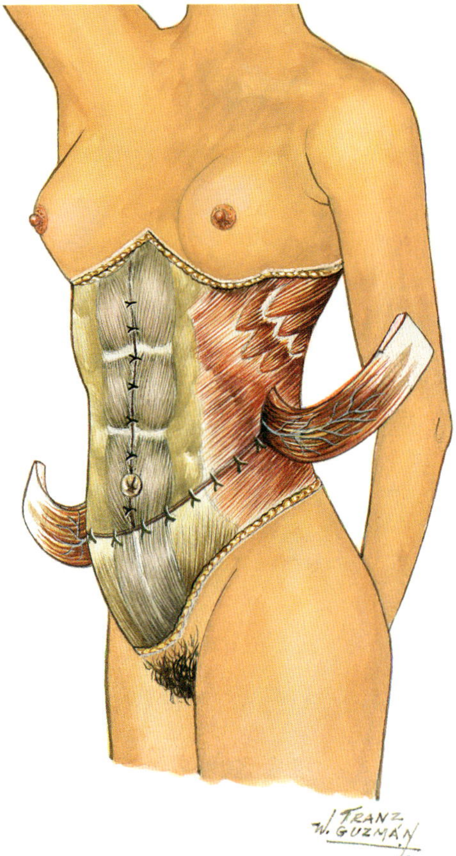

C

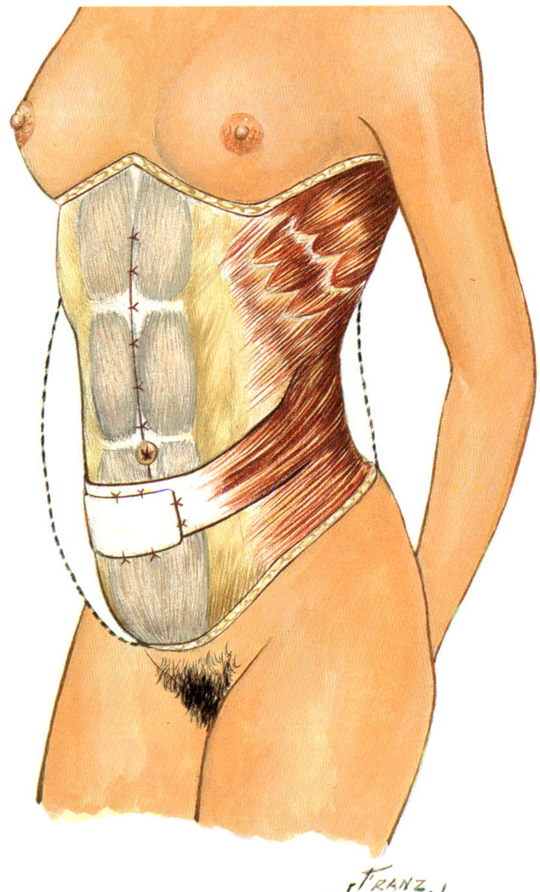

Figure 3 – 30. *(continued)*

D

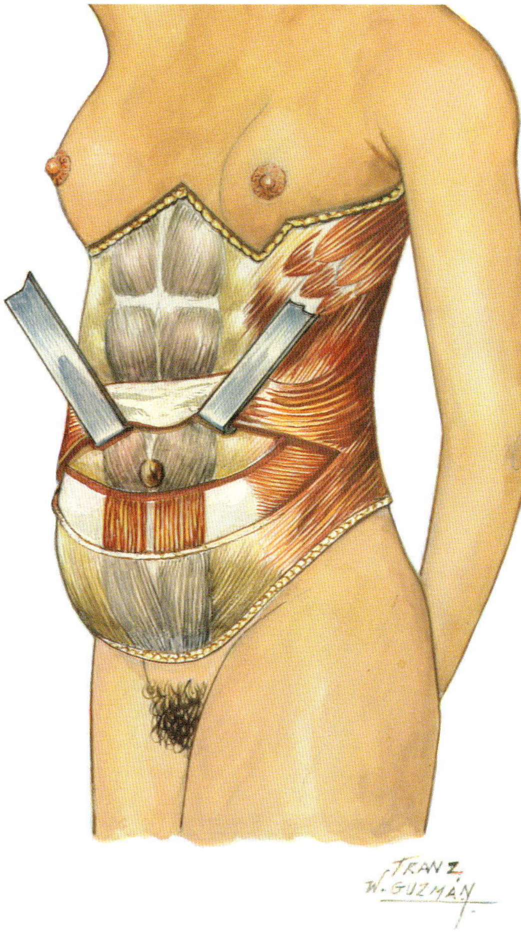

Figure 3-31. Schematic drawing of the girdle procedure without diastasis of the rectus muscles.

Type III: Delfino-Appiani

The Psillakis and Appiani techniques can be combined with the following procedure: the oblique muscle is separated from the external margin of rectus sheath, but a segment of 5 to 7 cm of the anterior rectus fascia is included, beginning 1.5 cm under the umbilicus (Figs. 3-32A-D, 3-33A-D).

THE NAVEL IN TYPE IV ABDOMINOPLASTY

In the type IV abdomen, to allow the plicature of the rectus muscles in the epigastric region, two techniques can be used: releasing and reinsertion of the navel or plication without detaching the navel.

If the first one is employed during the undermining of the abdominal flap, the umbilical stalk is incised transversely at the base near the fixation of the aponeurosis. Before we do this, it is important to confirm the fact that the patient has no umbilicus hernia, omphalocele, or fistula. The umbilicus scar remains attached to the abdominal flap and the dissection continues in the epigastric region (see Fig. 3-13). After plicature of the musculoaponeurotic layer and defatting of the subcutaneous tissue, the navel is reinserted at its original position or 1 to 2 cm lower if the navel was more than 15 cm from the pubis. For fixation of the navel, several stitches are placed between the aponeurosis and the dermis of the navel.

If we use the technique without detaching the navel, the stalk needs to be carefully isolated during the undermining (see Fig. 3-14A, B). With long fiberoptic illuminated retractors (see Fig. 3-12), the undermining can be done up to the inferior ribs and xiphoid. To perform the plicature of the rectus muscles, the first stitch is placed in the middle between the xiphoid and navel. The other stitches are more easily placed after the first one. The umbilicus stalk is shortened by anchoring the

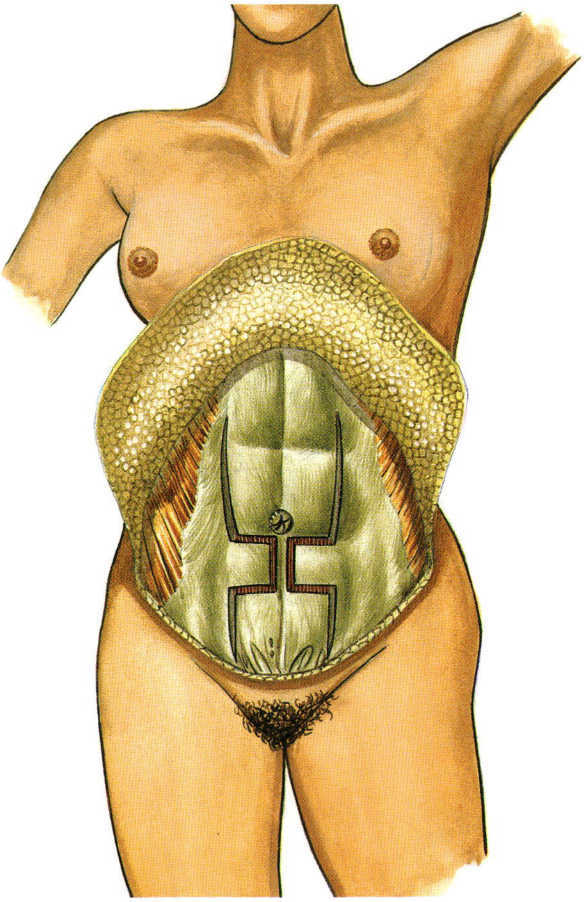

A

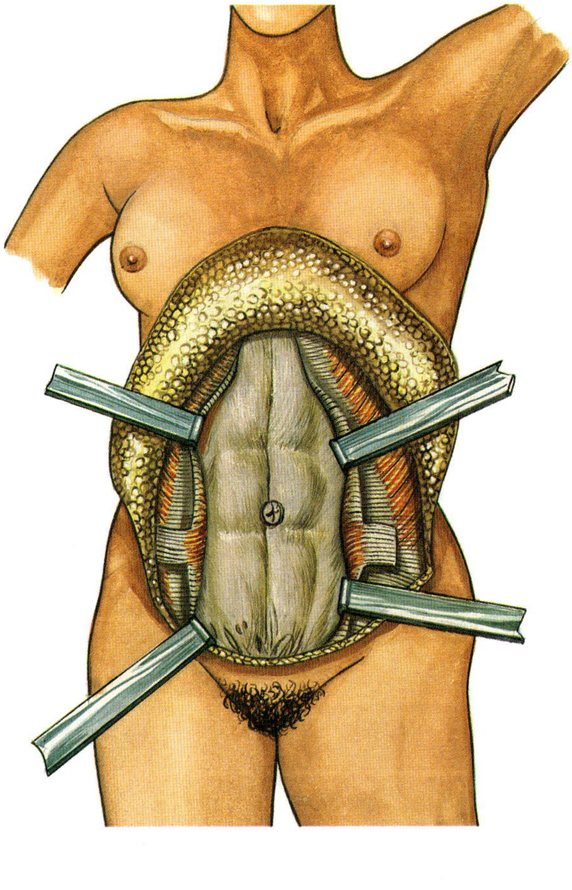

B

Figure 3–32. A–D: Schematic drawing of the combination of the Psillakis and Appiani techniques (Delfino). (Drawings by Franz W. Guzmán.) *(Figure continues)*

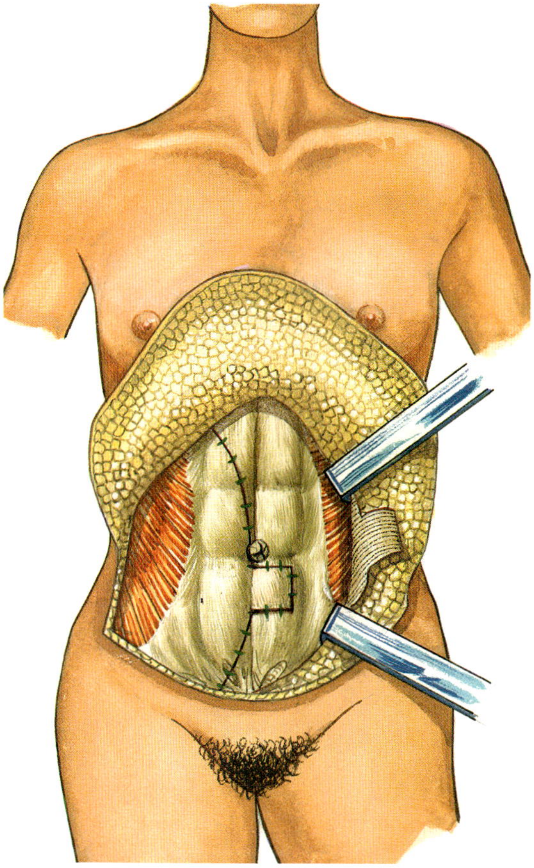

C

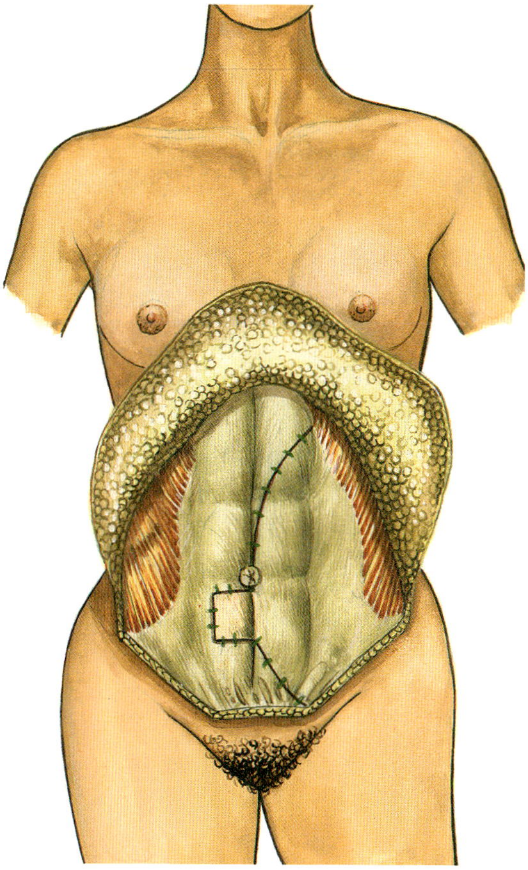

D

Figure 3–32. *(continued)*

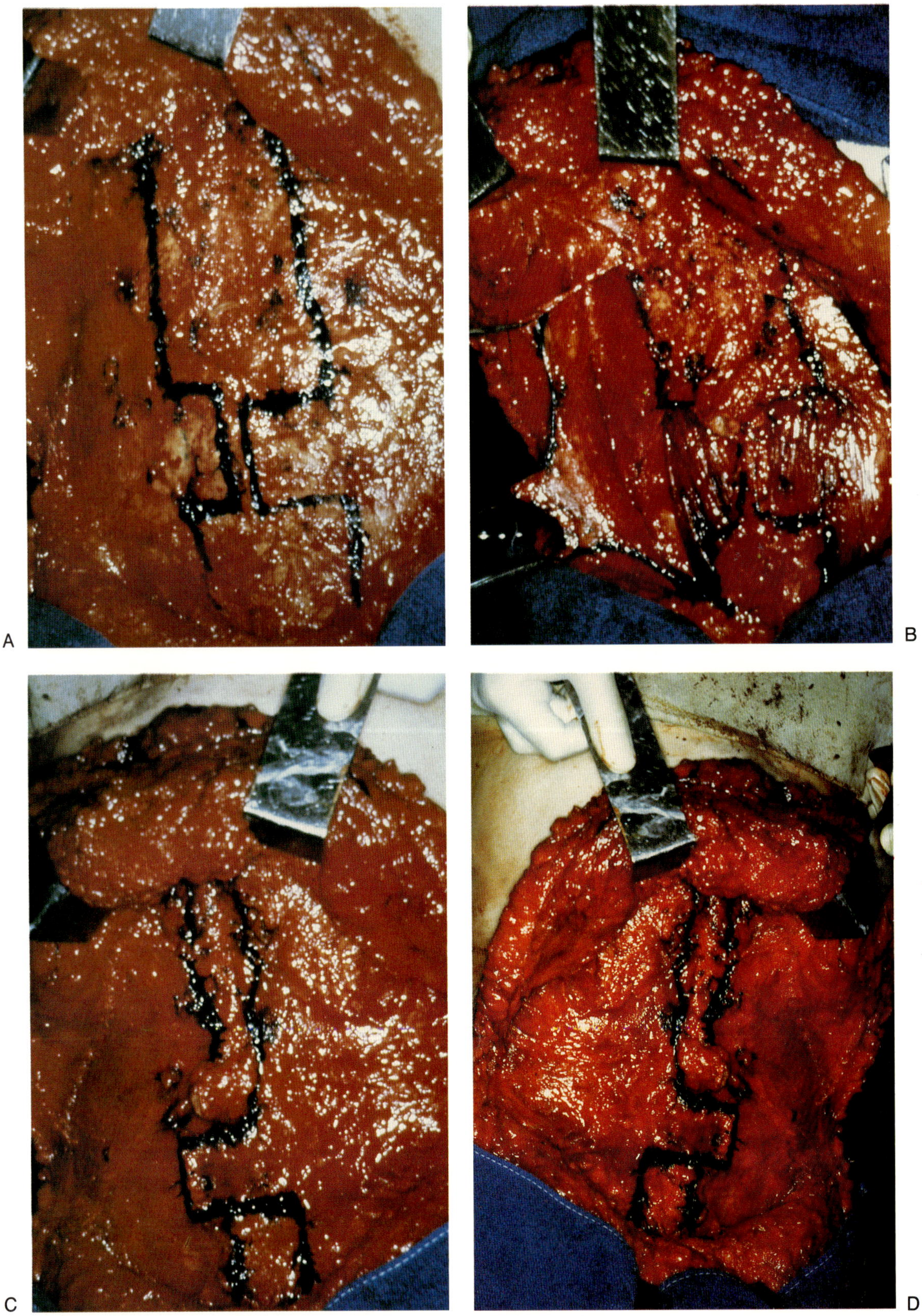

Figure 3–33. A–D: Intraoperative view of the dissection of the external oblique muscle, including a segment of the rectus sheath.

dermis to the anterior rectus sheath with separate stitches.

THE NAVEL IN TYPE V ABDOMINOPLASTY

In type V abdominoplasty, in order to build the navel, a U-shaped incision is made 15 mm in size, pedicled inferiorly (Figs. 3–34A–D, 3–35A–E).

The subcutaneous adipose tissue is removed in a cylinder shape to rebuild the anatomic depression around the umbilicus. The flap formed by the U incision is completely defatted and only skin remains. At the midpoint of the lower section of the remaining navel, an incision is made through its whole thickness, up to the proximity of aponeurosis where the U flap is sutured. After all the sutures are made, we can see that the traction of the skin flap at the base of the navel produces a natural depression that extends beyond the subumbilical area.

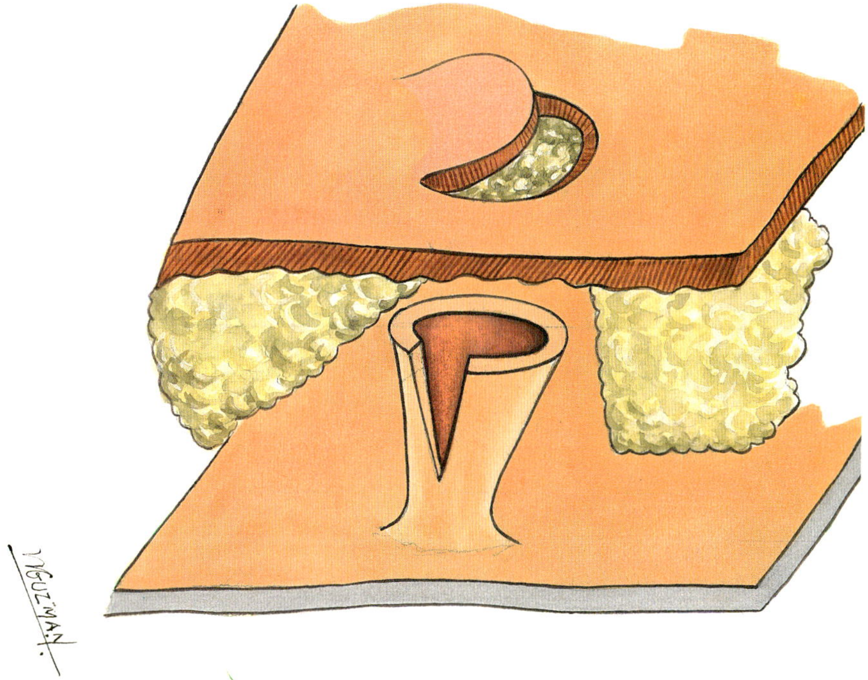

A

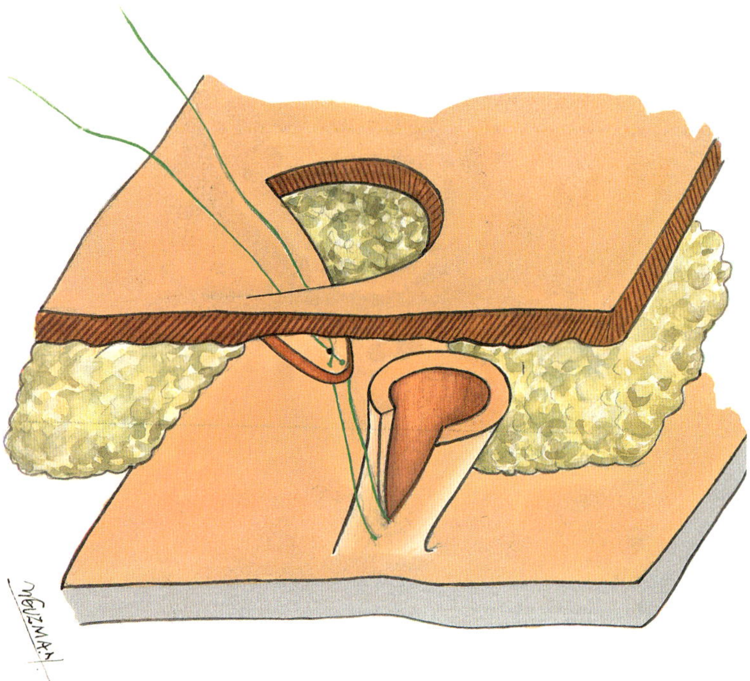

B

Figure 3–34. A–D: Schematic drawings of the repositioning of the navel on a type V abdomen. *(Figure continues)*

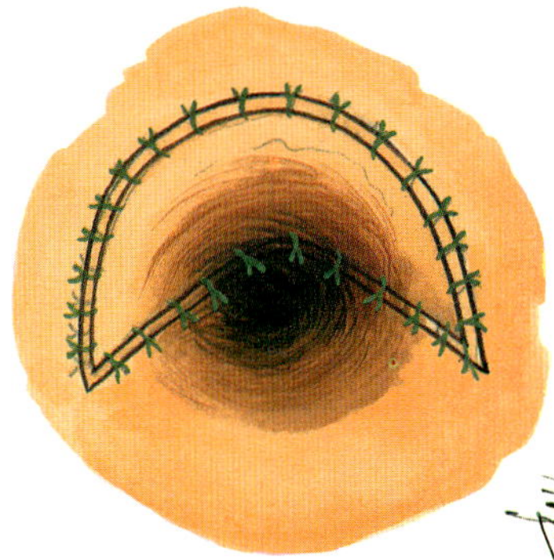

C

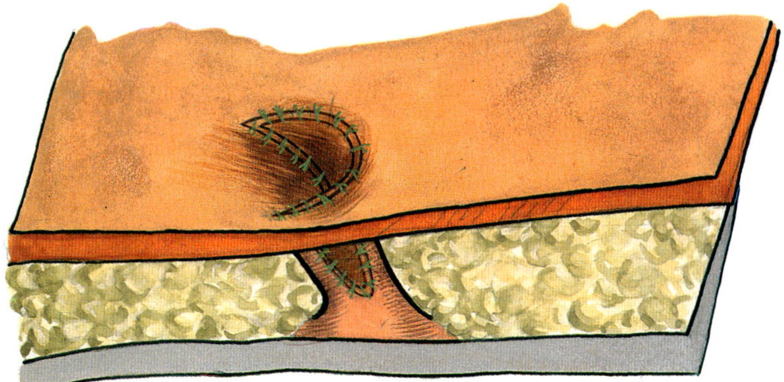

D

Figure 3–34. *(continued)*

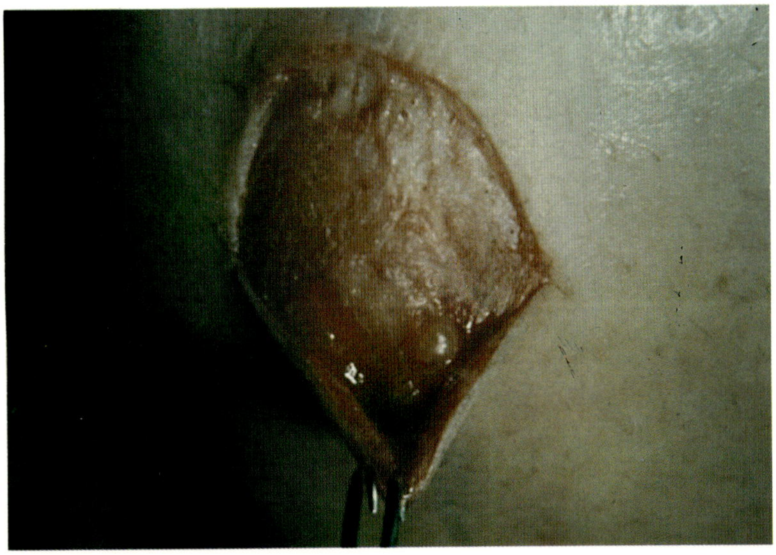

A

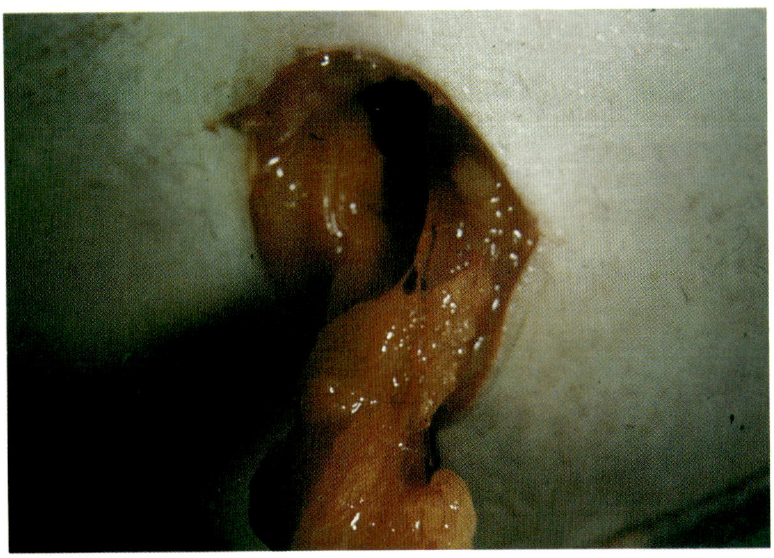

B

Figure 3–35. **A–E:** Intraoperative view of the repositioning of the navel. **A:** The U incision pedicled inferiorly; **B:** defatting of the subcutaneous tissue; **C:** the abdominal incision prepared to receive the navel; **D:** the navel is divided inferiorly where the "U" flap is sutured; **E:** the final natural aspect of the navel. *(Figure continues)*

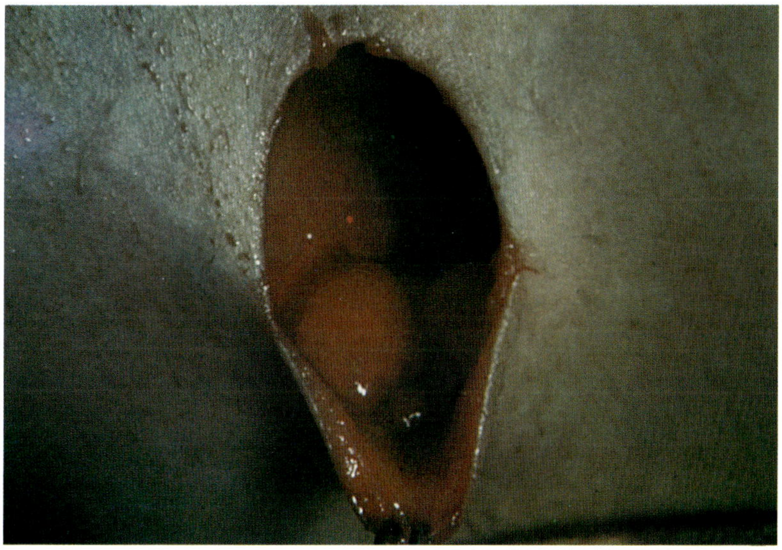

C

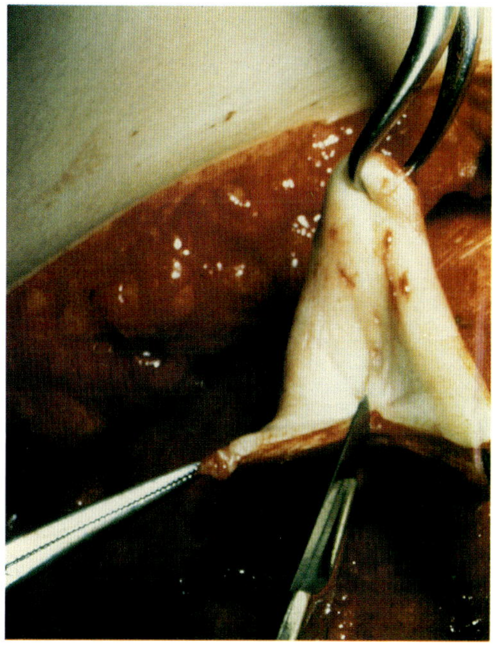

D

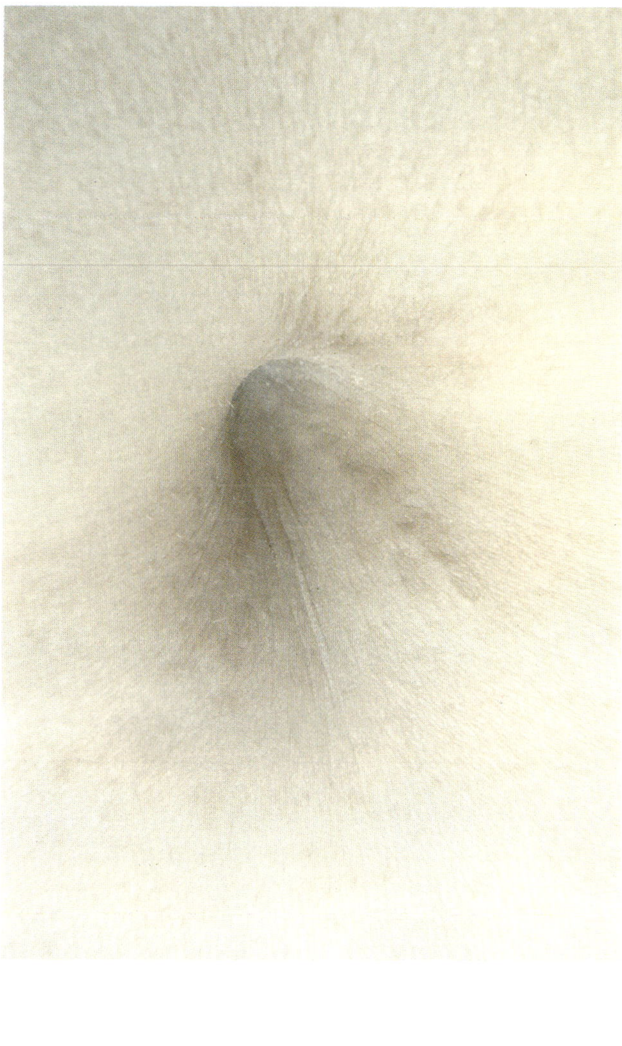

E

Figure 3-35. *(continued)*

RIB RESECTION TO CORRECT ASYMMETRIES OF THE UPPER ABDOMEN

During pregnancy, the augmentation of abdominal volume produces an outward and forward rotation of the ribs, increasing the inferior diameter of the thorax. After parturition, these alterations reverse but in some cases can remain an evident asymmetric projection of the inferior ribs. Some patients complain of the difference, requiring surgery for correction.

In the clinical examination a bulging area is seen in the superior epigastrium in one side due not only to the position of the ribs, but also due to hypertrophy of the rectus abdominis muscle that inserts over it. To improve this asymmetry, partial resection of the rib cartilage is performed (Fig. 3-36A-C). After we have completely undermined the abdominal flap, if we press the musculoaponeurotic layer near the inferior ribs, the area that needs treatment can be seen. A transverse incision is made with electrocautery in the anterior aponeurosis and in the muscle to expose the ribs, which are resected in segments in those areas that are most projected. To avoid damage to the pleura, the dissection needs to be carefully done in the posterior part of the periosteum and perichondrium: the cartilage and bone are resected in pieces. Results can be seen on Figure 3-37A, B and 3-38A, B.

SCULPTURE OF THE SUBCUTANEOUS TISSUE DEFATTING AREAS AND SAL

The sculpturing of the fat from the subcutaneous tissue is important so that the flap conforms to the new shape of the musculoaponeurotic layer and the abdomen is rebuilt in the "lyre form," which gives the abdomen its aesthetic appearance. This sculpturing is important to perform in all types of abdomens and can be obtained by liposuction and defatting with a knife.

In a type I abdomen, when only liposuction is used, depressions need to be created to rebuild the semilunar line and the midline over the rectus muscle and immediately under the umbilicus to maintain the lyre form. In types II to V abdominoplasty defatting can be done with SAL (Fig. 3-39A, B) or with the knife. Defatting with the knife is performed solely under the superficial fascia and is extended upward to the level of the umbilicus line in the direction of the ribs.

In types IV and V abdominoplasty, the medial sulcus in the epigastric region is rebuilt by the resection of a strip of fat and superficial fascia from the xiphoid to the new umbilicus (Fig. 3-40). This resection can be done by knife or open SAL. The resection of the superficial fascia breaks its continuity and will mold the skin over the musculoaponeurotic layer. If the superficial fascia is not divided, it will work as an armature under the skin because it is less elastic than the skin and will produce a protuberance in the epigastric region when the flap is pulled inferiorly.

In type V abdominoplasty the thickness at the inferior margin of the flap must be reduced to equalize the margins of the wound to avoid a bulging area immediately over the scar. The margin of the flap must be very thin (Fig. 3-41A, B), but special care must be taken not to destroy the blood supply; otherwise small areas of superficial necrosis will be produced.

To reduce the thickness of the flap, the fat under the Scarpa's fascia is resected with the knife up to 7 to 8 cm over the navel. Laterally, this resection is beveled in the flanks and in the hypochondrium to avoid damage to the vessels. Care must be taken not to damage the intercostal arteries.

Liposuction of the hips is frequently associated with abdominoplasty and gives a better contour to the trunk. In some cases where excess skin is present at the hips, the incision of type V abdominoplasty is extended to the posterior axillary line to resect it.

CUTANEOUS TISSUE TO BE RESECTED

The cutaneous tissue to be resected varies according to the excess skin each patient has and the type of abdomen. While minor resections from types II to IV are always within the limit of the inguinal line, resections in type V that extend up to the umbilicus surpass laterally the anterosuperior iliac spine. In extreme cases the incision reaches the posterior axillary line and in pathologic conditions may surround the trunk up to the lumbar region.

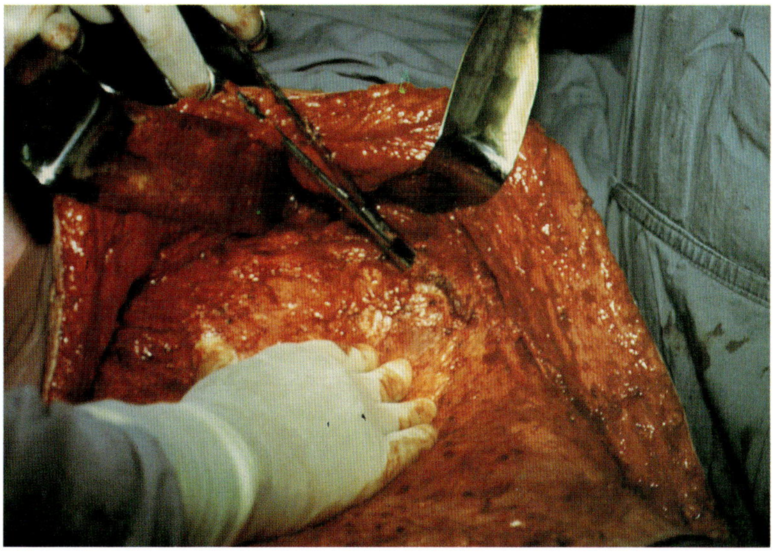

A

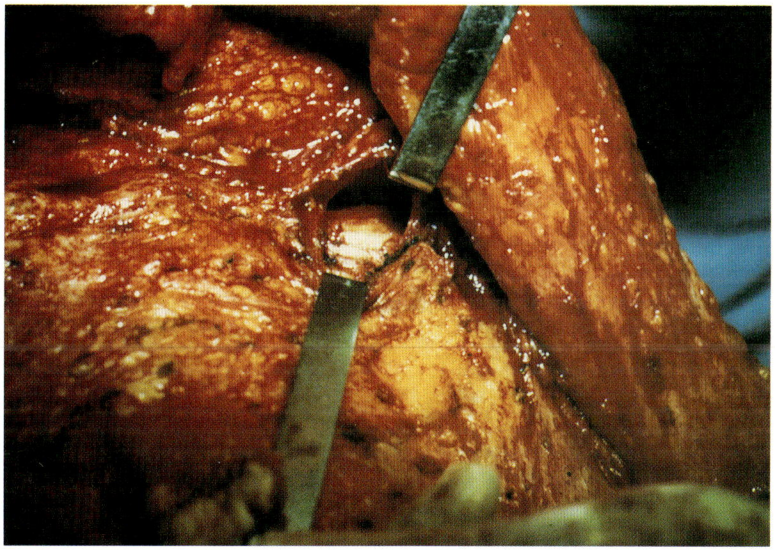

B

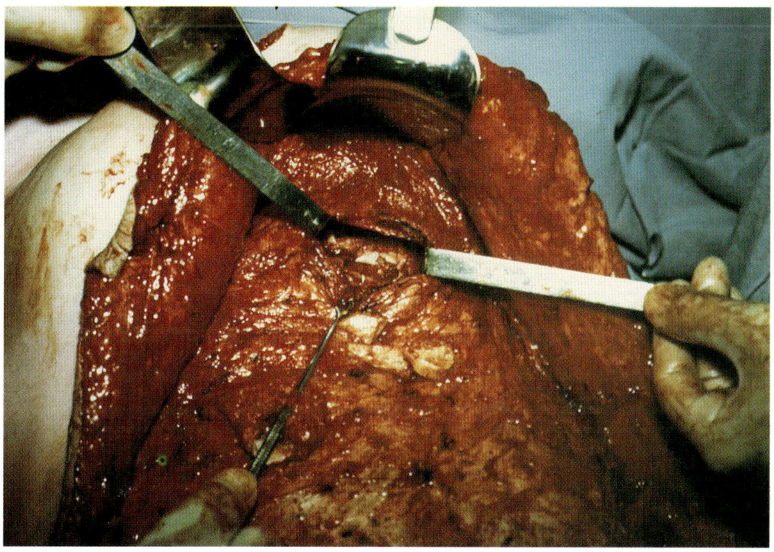

C

Figure 3-36. A-C: To improve asymmetries in the upper abdomen, partial resection of the rib cartilage is necessary. A: Pressing the musculoaponeurotic layer; B: transverse incision in the anterior sheath of the rectus abdominis muscle; C: the muscle is sectioned with electrocautery and the ribs are disected and removed in pieces.

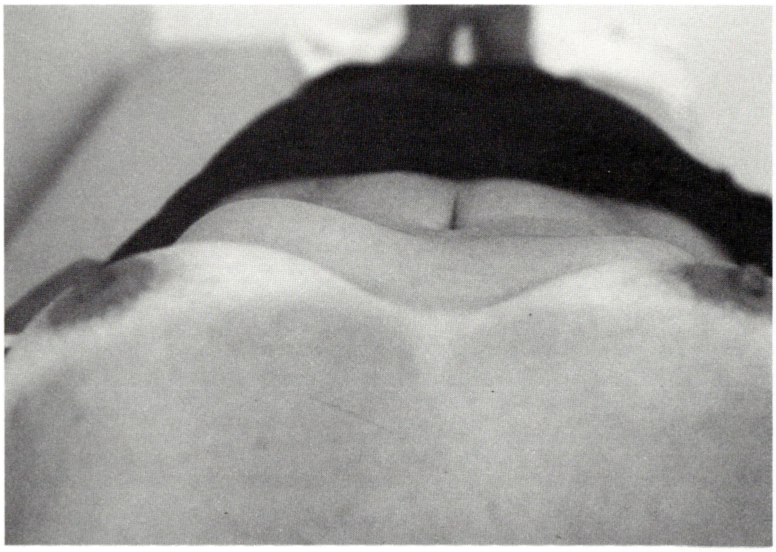

A

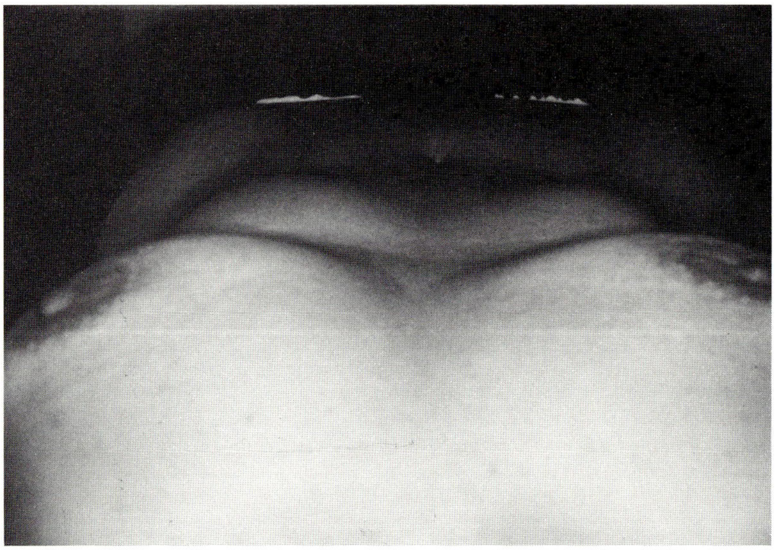

B

Figure 3-37. A: Patient with the left side more prominent than the right one. B: Result 1 year after rib resection.

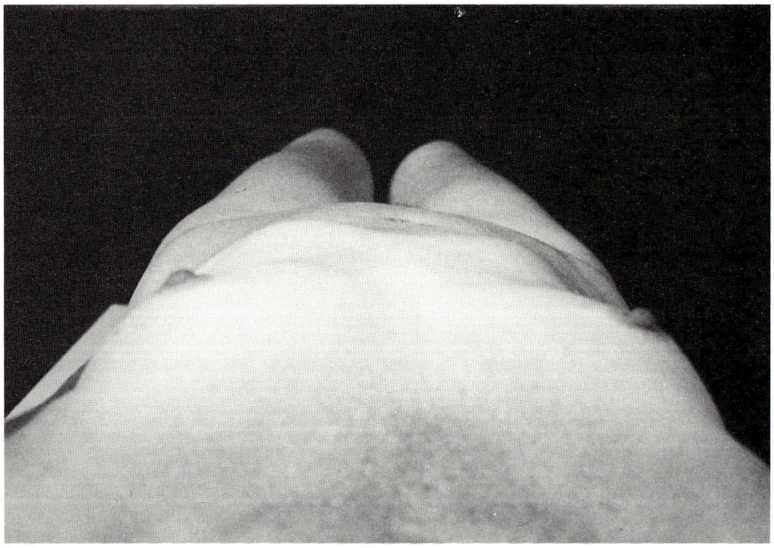

A

Figure 3-38. A: Left side prominent due to asymmetry of the ribs. B: Six-month postoperative result. *(Figure continues)*

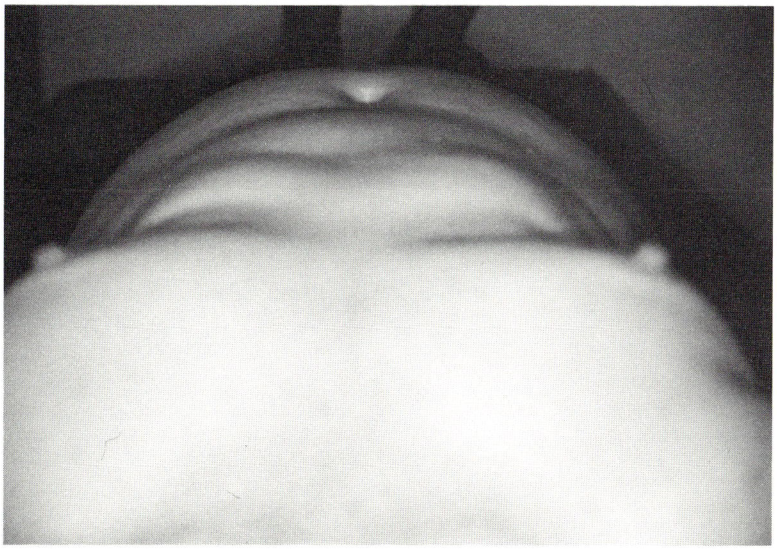

Figure 3–38. *(continued)* B

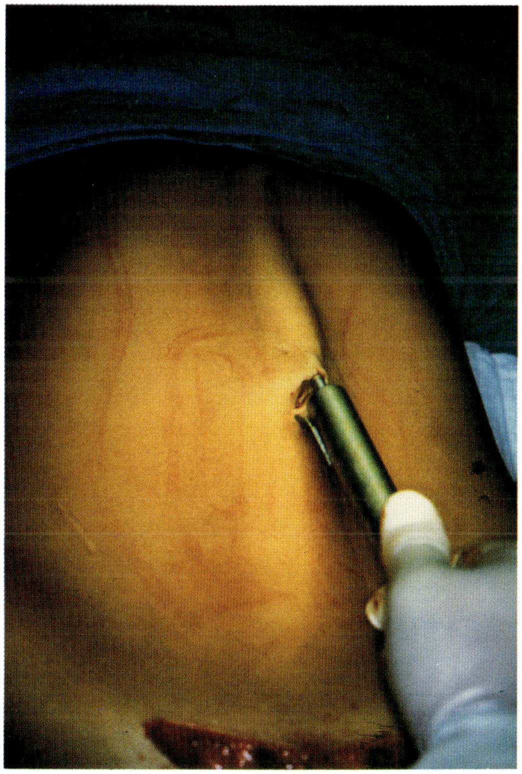

A

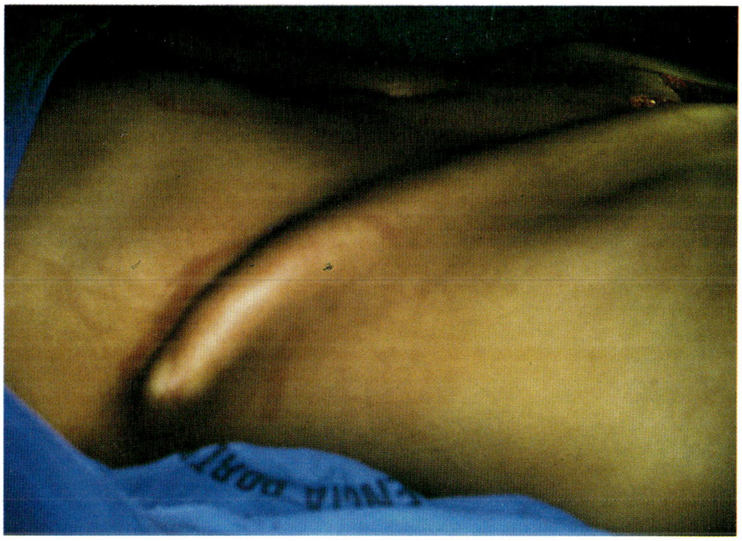

B

Figure 3–39. A, B: Sculpture of the subcutaneous tissue can be done by suction-assisted lipectomy: to rebuild the medial sulcus of the superior abdomen (A) and to reduce the waist (B).

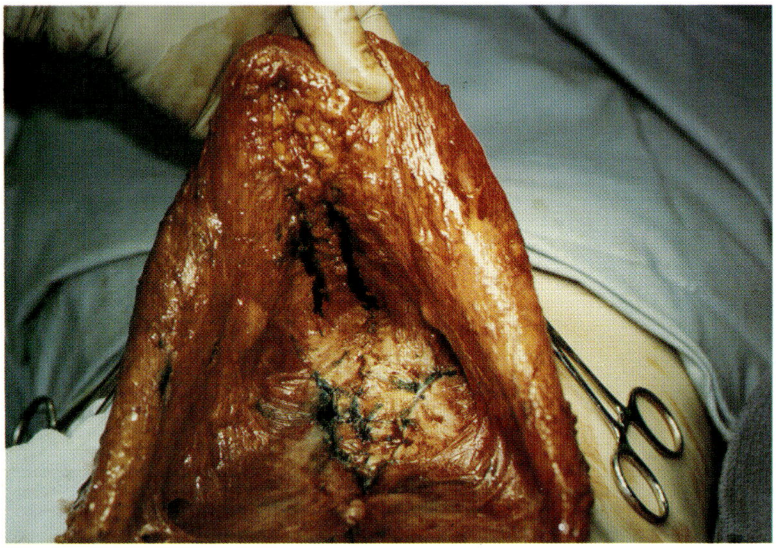

Figure 3-40. The medial sulcus is also rebuilt in types IV and V abdominoplasty by resecting a strip of superficial fascia and fat with the knife.

A

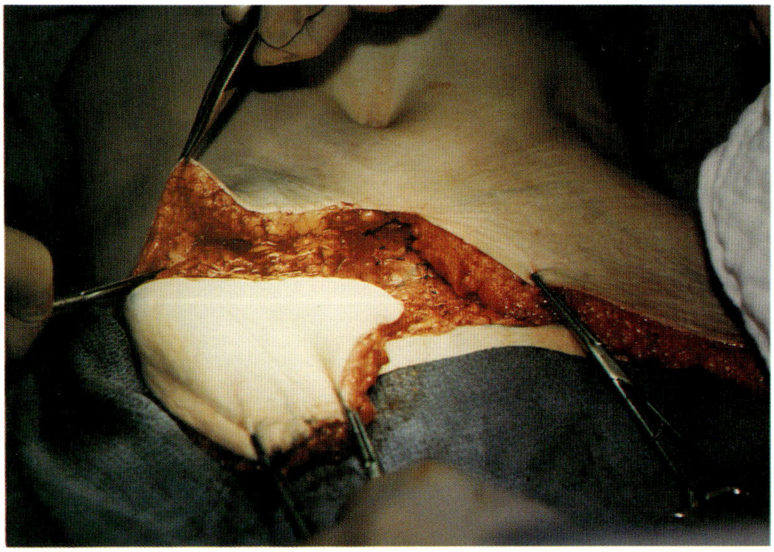

B

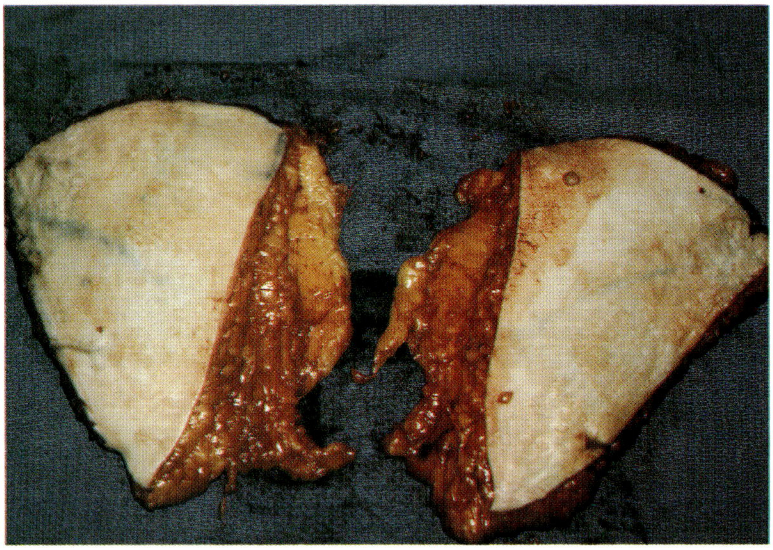

Figure 3-41. A, B: In the inferior margin of the flap the thickness is reduced with the knife to equalize the margin of the wound.

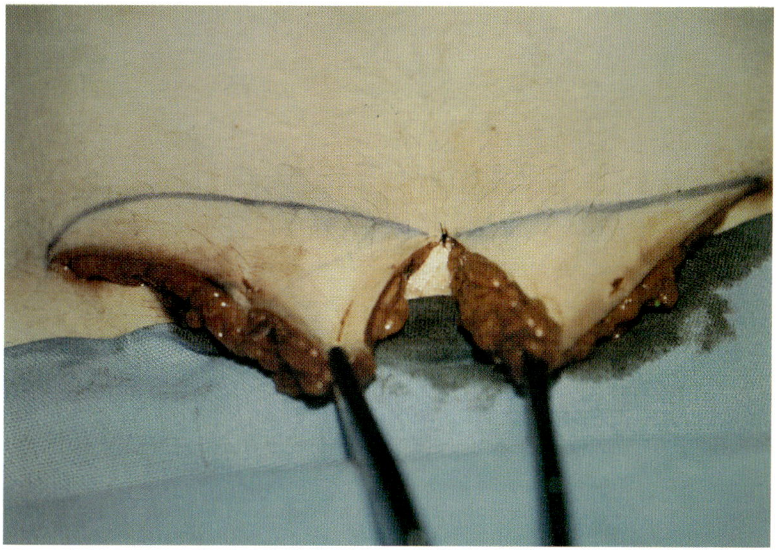

A

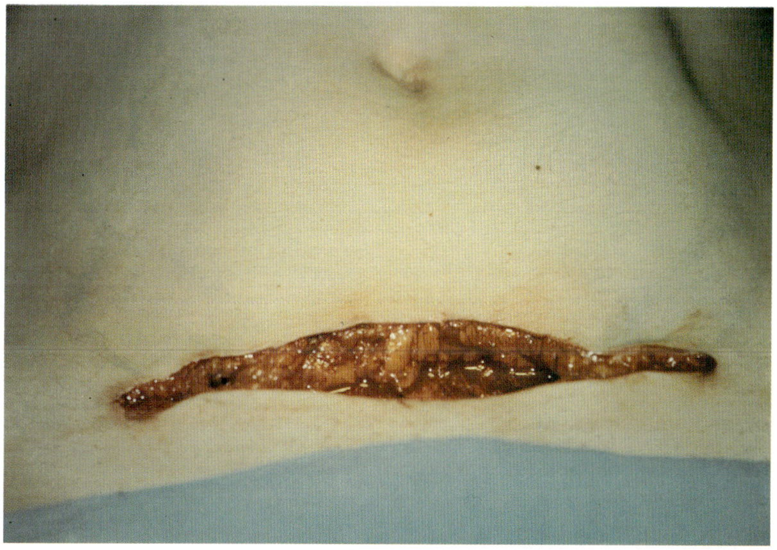

B

Figure 3–42. A, B: In types II to IV, to calculate the quantity of skin to be resected, the flap is divided and a stitch is placed and two lateral triangles are resected.

In types II and III, to calculate the quantity of skin to resect, the flap is slightly stretched downward and divided in the midline; a stitch is placed at this point and the two lateral triangles are resected (Fig. 3–42A, B). We emphasize that the flap must be pulled slightly medially to avoid "dog ears" on the extremities of the wound. In type IV, the procedure and details are similar, but with greater cutaneous resection.

In type V abdominoplasty the flap is divided in the midline up to the navel during dissection. At the end of the surgery, after the navel is relocated, the flap is pulled medially (Figs. 3–43A,B, 3–44A, B) to obtain the best modeling. A stitch affixes the flap to the pubis before the excess tissue is resected. The resection can be done in two pieces or in four pieces (Fig. 3–45A–C).

In type VI the flap is divided in the middle to determine the amount to be resected and a stitch is located at the level of the sternum. We resect two triangles laterally or we use part of the flap for breast augmentation (Fig. 3–46A, B).

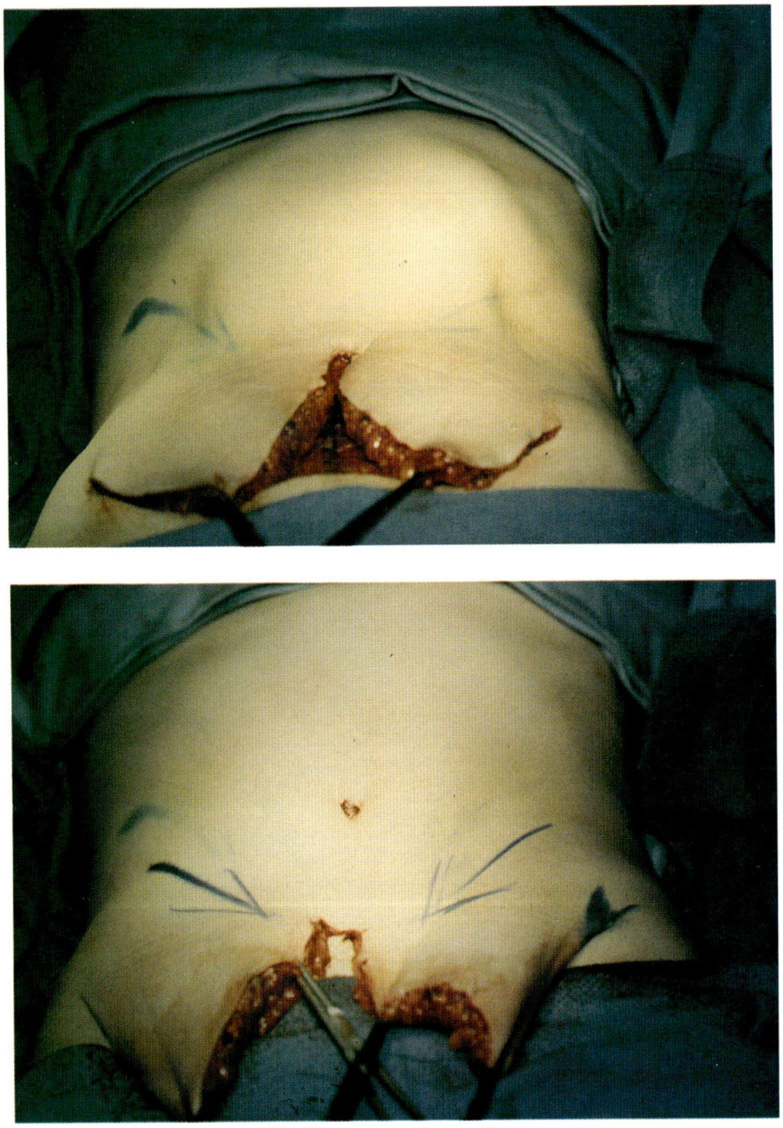

A

B

Figure 3-43. A, B: Direction that the flap needs to be pulled to avoid "dog ears."

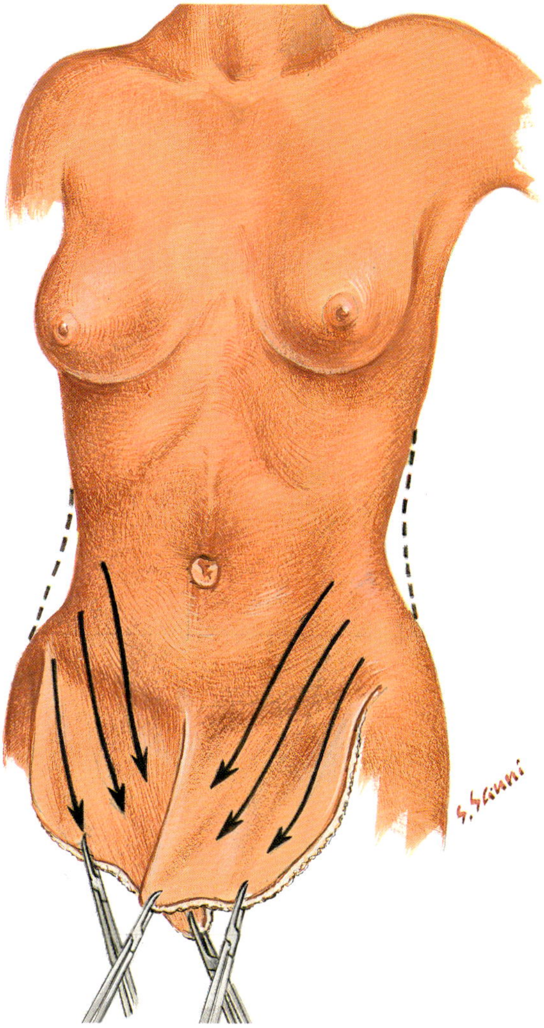

A

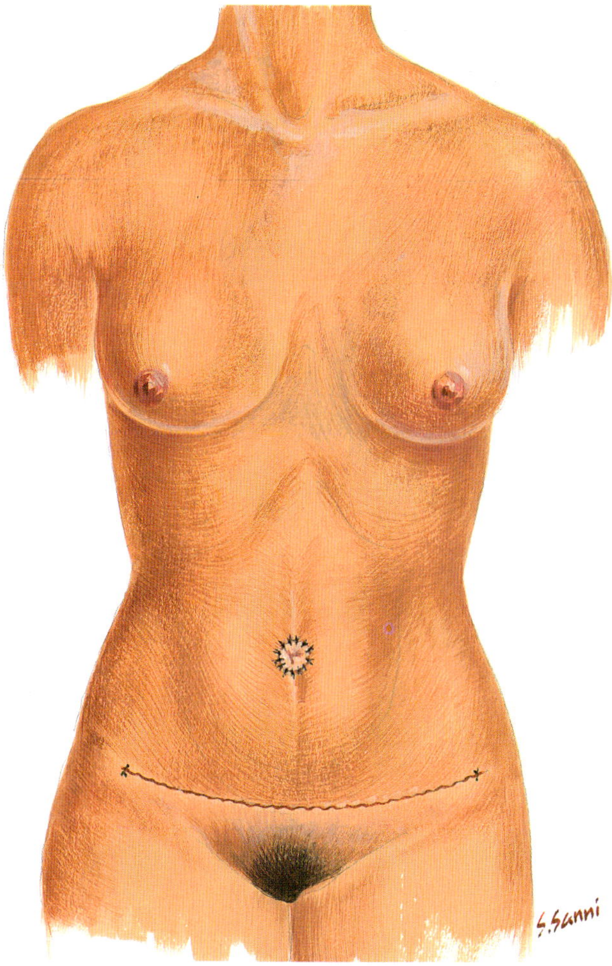

B

Figure 3–44. A, B: Schematic drawing to indicate the direction the flaps must be pulled to shape the abdomen better.

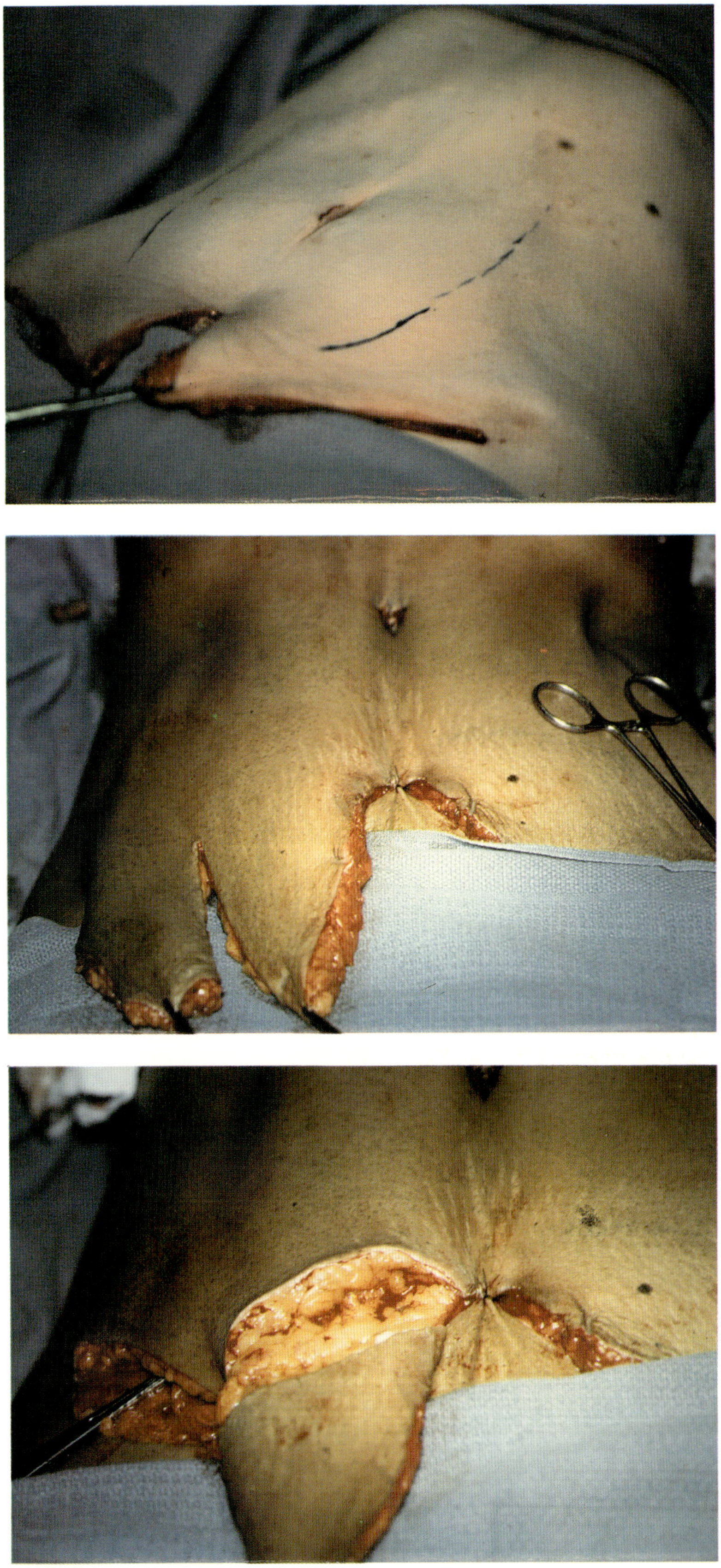

A

B

C

Figure 3–45. A–C: In type V the flaps are pulled medially and a stitch is placed in the middle of the pubis. The excess of cutaneous tissue is resected in two pieces or in four pieces by dividing each of the flaps in the middle.

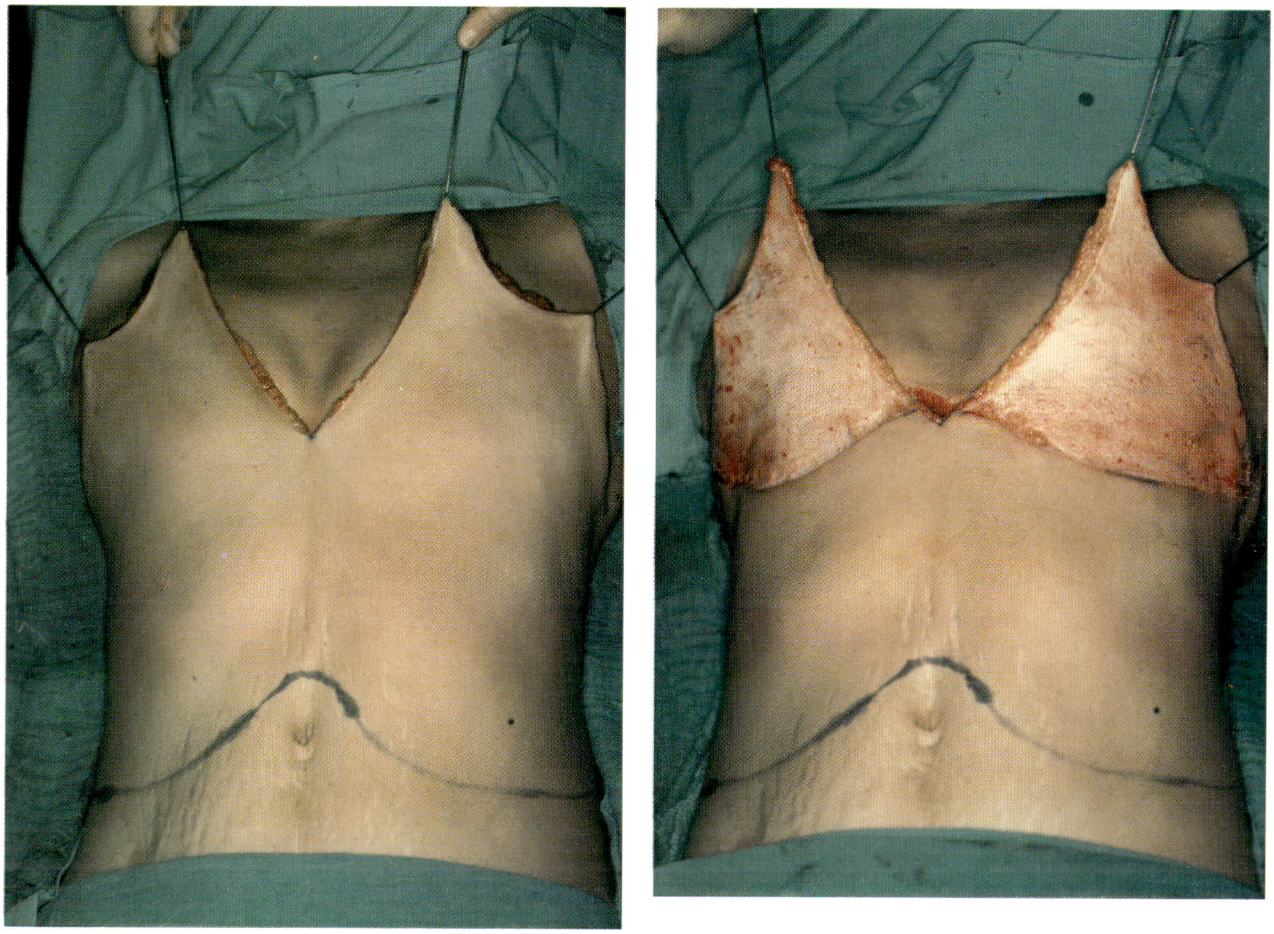

A B

Figure 3–46. A, B: In type VI the flap is divided to determine the amount to be resected. The flap can also be used for breast augmentation.

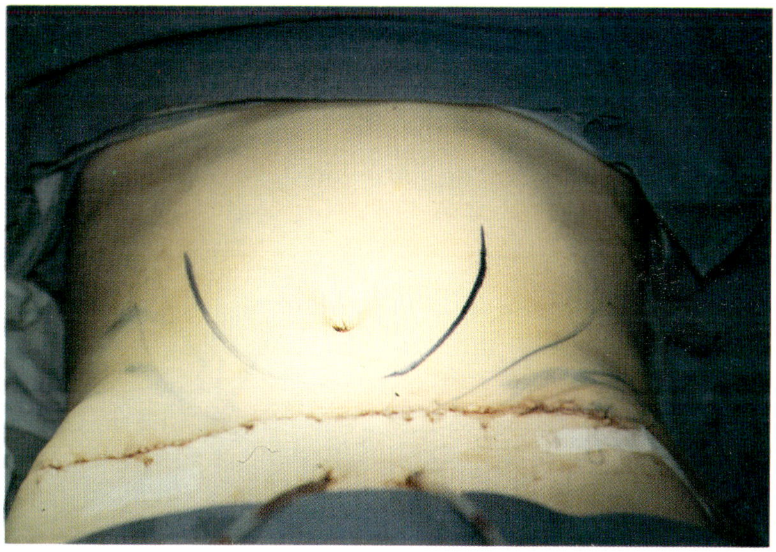

Figure 3–47. Two suction drains extending from the xiphoid to the pubis exteriorized by a stab incision in the pubis.

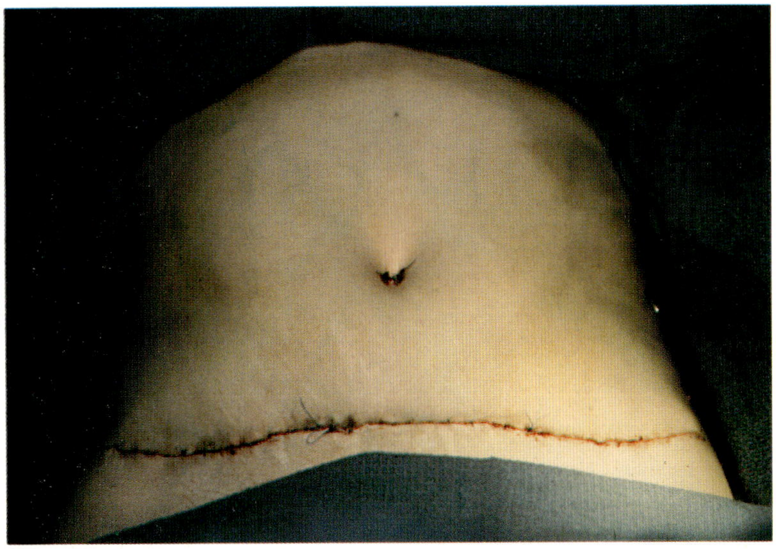

Figure 3–48. The wound is closed in layers with a final running subcuticular suture.

A

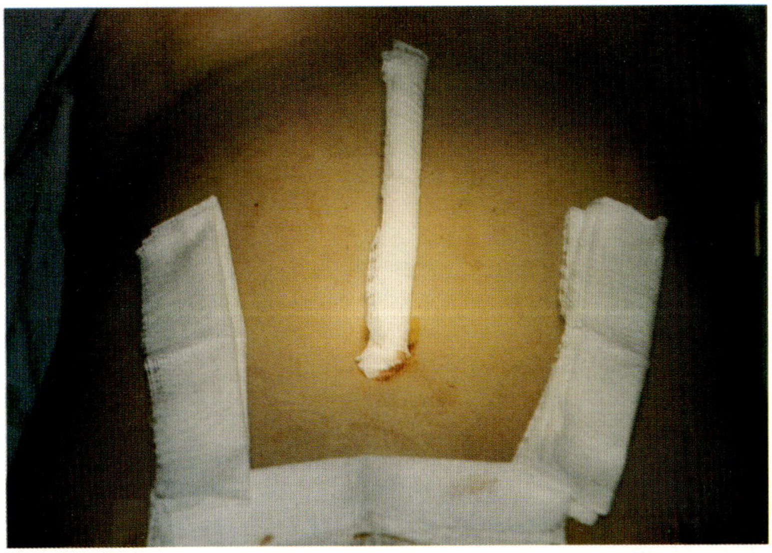

B

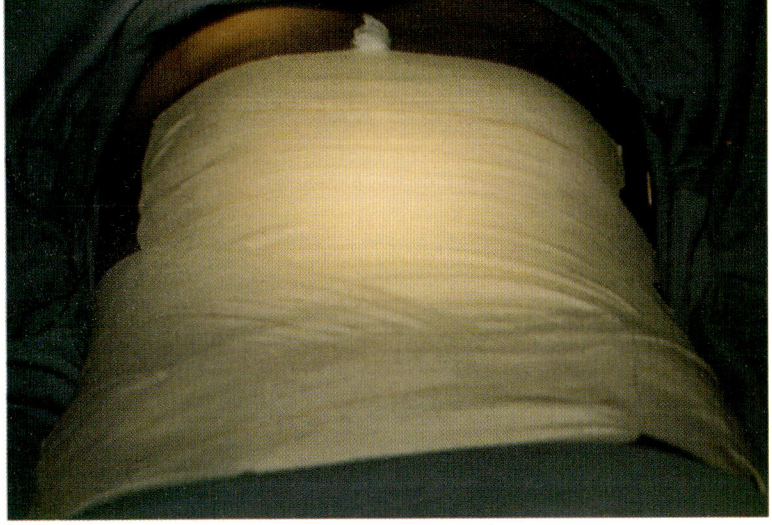

Figure 3–49. A, B: A cylinder of sponges from the xiphoid to the navel shapes the depression of the medial sulcus; compressive elastic bandages are used to immobilize the flap.

DRAINS

Drains are routinely used in surgeries of types IV and V. Two suction drains are used, extending vertically from the xiphoid to the pubis with a stab incision on the pubis. They are maintained routinely for 24 to 48 hours. In cases in which we associate abdominoplasty with the resection of large quantities of fat by SAL, drains are maintained for 5 or more days (Fig. 3–47).

SUTURE

The suture of the wound needs to be done in two layers: at the subcutaneous tissue and dermis, finishing with a running subcuticular suture to obtain the best possible scar (Fig. 3–48). We prefer to use nylon in all layers instead of absorbable material.

DRESSING

Compressive elastic bandages are used in order to compress and immobilize the abdomen completely. For this purpose, elastic tape is used in transverse and oblique directions crossing in the midline. To shape the depression of the medial sulcus on the epigastrium, we use a cylinder of sponges from the xiphoid to the navel for a week (Fig. 3–49A, B). The dressing is first changed after 24 hours and, up to the 7th day it is again changed twice, depending on cleanliness. Over the dressing, the patient may wear a girdle not only to help the compression, but also to allow the patient to feel psychologically more confident.

4

Postoperative Period

IMMEDIATE POSTOPERATIVE ROUTINE

We assist the patient in becoming ambulatory 24 hours after surgery. The ingestion of food is carefully supervised with normalization of peristalsis of the bowels. Abdominal distension can produce pain, discomfort, and dehiscence of the musculoaponeurotic sutures. In patients with associated intra-abdominal surgery, the convenience of the use of a gastric tube needs to be analyzed. On singular instances of abdominoplasty, medication for gas relief may be given. Antibiotics are used only in cases in which the abdominoplasty was associated with liposuction or with intra-abdominal surgery.

Patients with types I to III abdominoplasty can leave the hospital in 24 hours and those with types IV and V, after 48 hours.

Stitches are removed after the 7th day and a girdle is maintained for 2 weeks. The patient can return to work after 2 weeks and perform normal exercises after 4 weeks. Exercises for the abdomen are encouraged after the fourth week, and the patient is followed up to 1 year after the operation for examination of the scar and shape of the abdomen.

COMPLICATIONS AND HOW TO AVOID THEM

Complications are not frequent in the hands of experienced and careful surgeons. The most frequent complication is seroma, especially in patients in whom SAL is associated with abdominoplasty and in obese patients. To avoid seromas, some measures can be taken: a very careful hemostasis is performed progressively during the elevation of the abdominal flap; gentle manipulation of the fat tissue; maintenance of the suction drains up to the day drainage is reduced to 35 cc. The incidence of seromas is proportionate to the amount of fat in the cutaneous tissue and to the trauma over it. Aggressive maneuvers in the undermining of the flap, excessive burn by electrocautery, and liposuction are the main causes of seromas, which are seen in the second postoperative week. The diagnosis is made when spontaneous drainage through the suture line occurs or by a localized distension of the abdominal wall. If the seroma is in the infraumbilical area, drainage is maintained through the incision. If it is localized in the upper abdomen, a transcutaneous puncture with needle is better treatment. Recurrence will occur three or four times and puncture needs to be repeated. Culture of the liquid can be performed for antibiotic intake.

Hematomas are less frequent than seromas and will also depend on the same measures taken to avoid seromas. As a preventive measure, prior to surgery, it is important to suspend the intake of medications that can increase bleeding. If a large hematoma occurs, it is important to remove it immediately to avoid the possibility of a consumption coagulopathy that will need treatment by transfusion and heparin. We had two cases of late hematomas due to sexual relations before the 15th day. These hematomas were produced by direct trauma to the infraumbilical area where the skin has no sensibility. For this reason, sexual relations are recommended only after 3 weeks, with care.

Necrosis of the skin can occur in several degrees and for several reasons. Small areas of necrosis of 1 to 2 cm can occur at the margin of the flap at the suture line due to excessive trauma by surgical instruments or by electrocautery (Fig. 4–1A, B). Small areas of skin loss can occur immediately over the umbilicus due to excessive defatting and tension at the suture of the superior margin of the flap to the navel that was fixed to the aponeurosis. Large areas of necrosis can occur in the suprapubic area in a triangular shape that may reach the umbilicus (Fig. 4–2A–F). This necrosis occurs due to tension, for several reasons: when the original position of the umbilicus was over 15 cm from the pubis and the abdominal flap was sutured in the pubis with tension; when a stitch was placed at the subcutaneous tissue between the pubis, the flap, and the rectus fascia at the same time with the intention of avoiding the elevation of the pubis; if the patient in the first few days of the postoperative period extends the trunk, the flap will be pulled in a superior direction and tension will occur with possible necrosis; the presence of vertical scars due to previous intra-abdominal surgeries; and excessive undermining of the abdominal flap in the superior abdomen dividing the perforators from

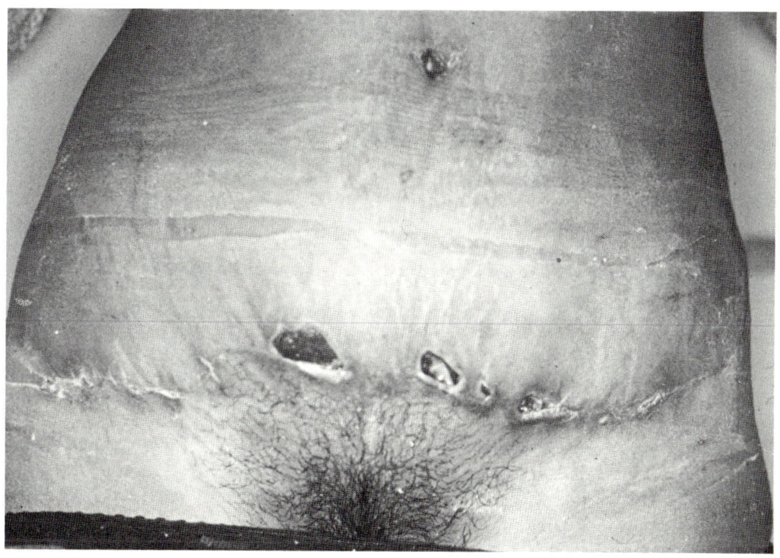
A

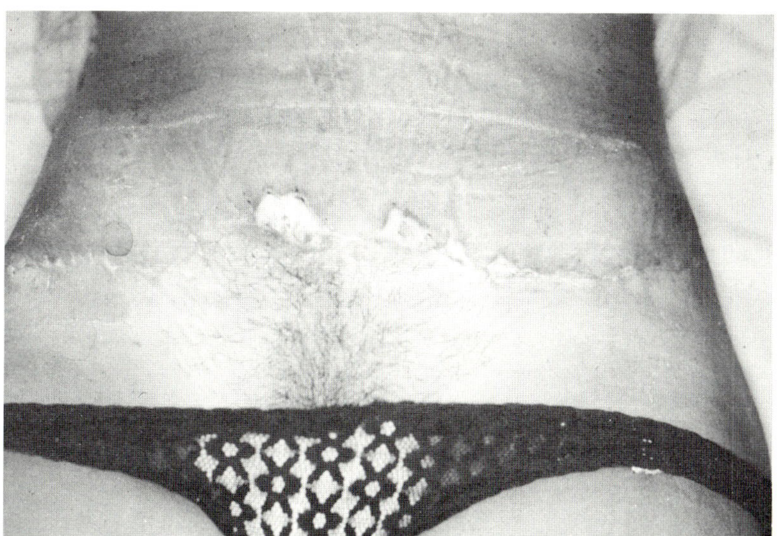
B

Figure 4–1. A, B: Complication: Small areas of necrosis can occur due to excessive trauma by electrocautery or surgical instruments.

A 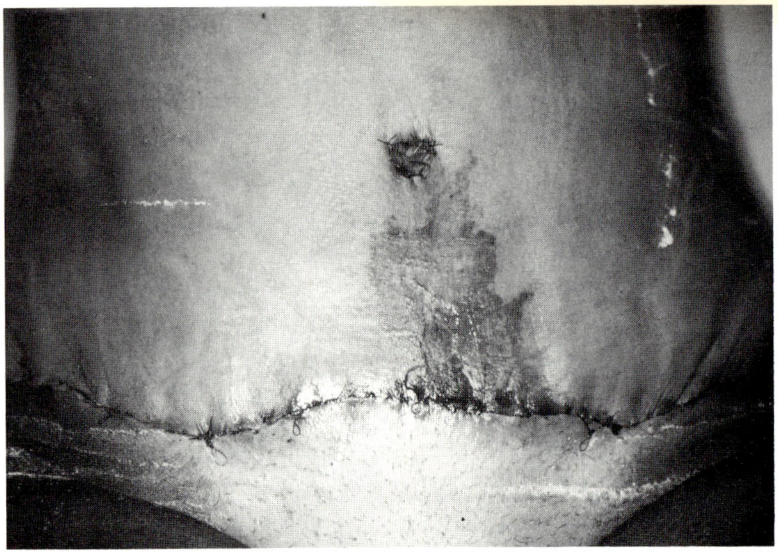

B 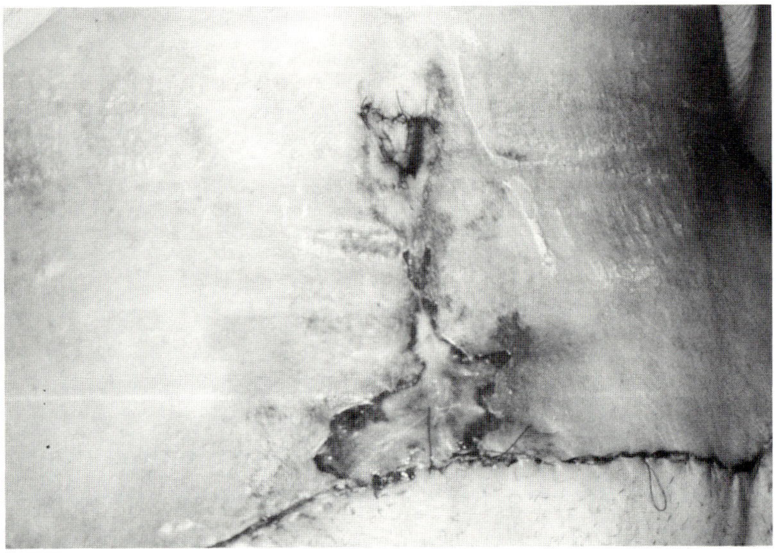

C 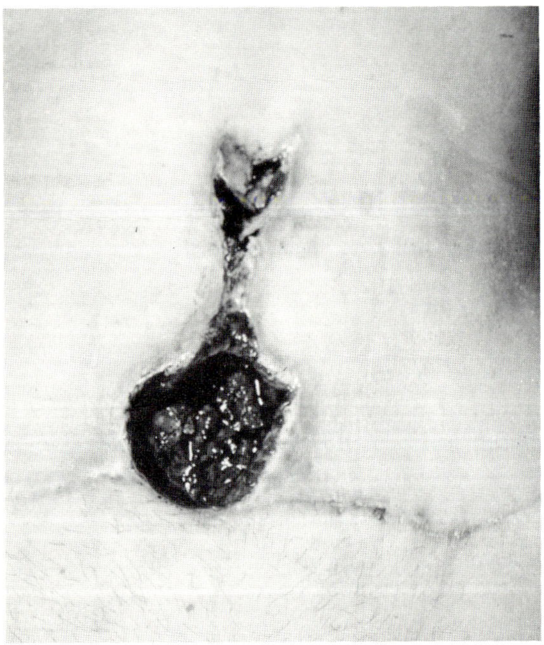

Figure 4–2. A–F: Complication: Large necrosis can occur due to tension in the suprapubic area; after the p.ɔcess is limited, reoperation is required to resect the necrotic area and a final inverted "T" scar remains. *(Figure continues)*

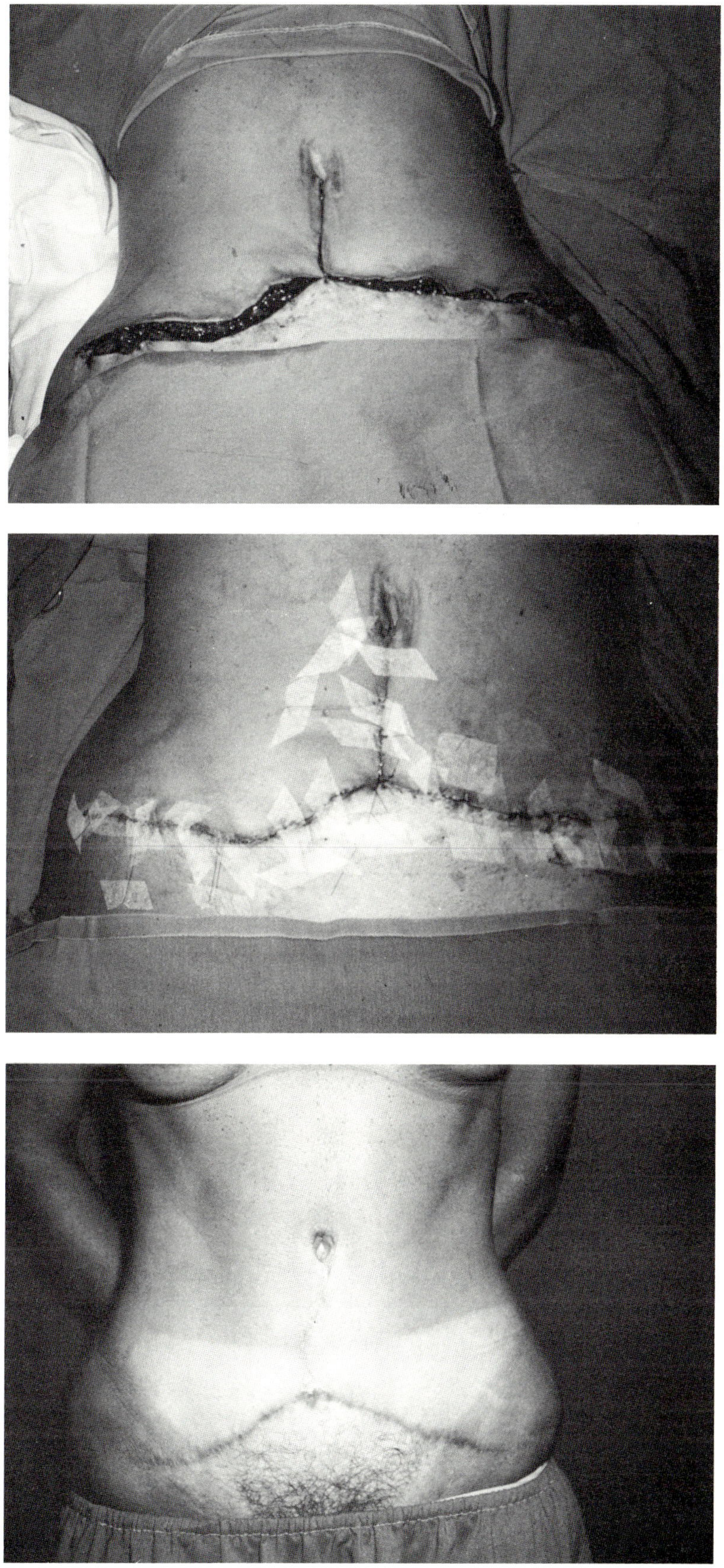
D
E
F

Figure 4–2. *(continued)*

the epigastric vessels. In this case the flap will act as a random flap with a high risk of necrosis. Treatment sometimes necessitates a skin graft that can be partially or totally resected later. Today, with the classification of the abdomen, the risk of necrosis is very low.

Primary infection is rare as a complication, but can occur secondary to small necrosis to tissue, to reaction to the stitches, and to hematomas. Treatment is performed by drainage, debridement of the necrotic tissue, and irrigation. Infection can occur in patients with low resistance, beginning in the suture line or in other areas and spreading over all the abdomen. In this case the patient must be taken to the operating room, the flap elevated, the wound thoroughly cleaned, and the dead tissue carefully debrided. Drainage for continuous irrigation is installed and large doses of intravenous antibiotics are used.

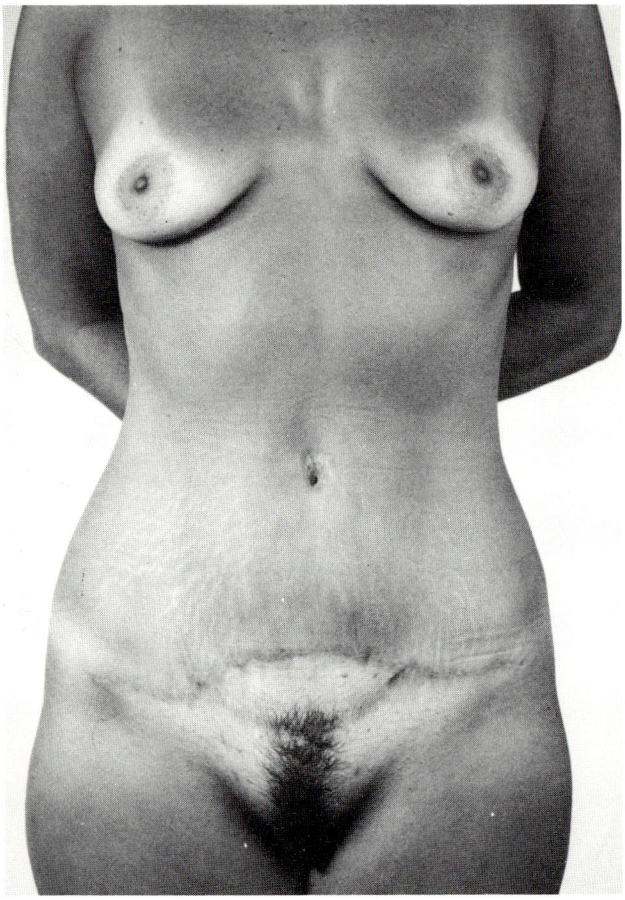

Figure 4–4. Elevation of the pubis with stretching of the vulva, that was very common before we introduced the classification system. The mistake occurs because of the excess of skin resection.

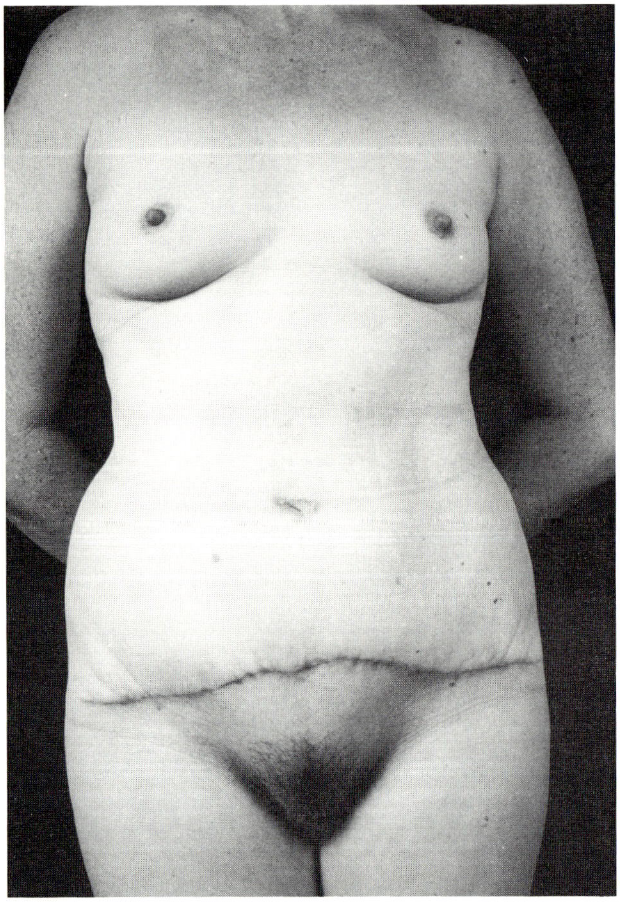

Figure 4–3. Asymmetry of the final scar due to technical mistakes.

Pulmonary embolism can occur less frequently with single abdominoplasty and more frequently when combined with gynecologic surgery. The use of pneumatic stockings can prevent this complication, which is secondary to the venous embolism of the legs. Treatment of this complication will not be discussed here, since it is well described in the literature.

Hypertrophic scars and keloids can occur and are more common around the navel. This happens in those techniques that use a round final scar to rebuild the navel in type V abdomens that with the constriction of the scar reduce the aperture of the navel, impeding its cleanliness. For the treatment of those scars, intense postoperative massage, injections of corticoids, and finally surgical revision with some type of plasty is used. Asymmetries of the scar may occur due to a technical mistake (Fig. 4–3).

The elevation of the pubis with secondary stretching of the vulva can occur in excessive cutaneous resection and is difficult to correct (Fig. 4–4).

Albeit abdominoplasty appears to be an easy procedure, it is not, and undesirable complications or unpleasant aesthetic results can occur in the hands of inexperienced surgeons. To avoid them, careful preoperative evaluation, gentle management of the tissue during surgery, good knowledge of the anatomy with emphasis on the blood supply, knowledge of the cause of complications, and sensitivity to aesthetics are important to put your conscience at ease if surprises occur.

QUESTIONS FREQUENTLY ASKED BY PATIENTS

Q: Will I feel pain after the operation?

A: The operation will produce some discomfort and some pain in movements, but pain medication will be prescribed.

Q: Can I die in surgery due to the anesthesia?

A: The risk always exists, but modern anesthesia is highly safe and you are in good health.

Q: What is the length of the operations?

A: Two to 3 hours.

Q: How long must I stay in the hospital?

A: Twenty-four hours for minor abdominoplasty and 48 hours for major ones.

Q: Do I have to diet?

A: No.

Q: How long will I need to be in a flexed position?

A: Approximately 1 week, in type V abdomen.

Q: How long will the swelling last?

A: The swelling will disappear progressively, but it will last up to the third month.

Q: When will the stitches be removed?

A: In 7 to 10 days.

Q: When will I be able to work?

A: After 2 weeks.

Q: When will I be able to resume exercises?

A: After 4 weeks.

Q: When will the sensation under the umbilicus return?

A: It will return progressively over 6 months.

Bibliography

Appiani E. Muscular plastic for aesthetic conformation of abdominal girdle. Transactions of the VIII International Congress of Plastic Surgery, 1983, Montreal: McGill University.

Appiani E. Muscular plastic for aesthetic conformation of abdominal girdle. Ann Plast Surg 13:97, 1984.

Appiani E. The use of the internal and transverse muscle and its limitations in abdominoplasty. XVI International Symposium of Plastic and Aesthetic Surgery. Institute of Plastic Surgery, Guadalajara, Mexico, 1988.

Ashbell TS. Abdominoplasty and combined procedure. Plast Reconstr Surg 79:316, 1987.

Avelar JM. Fat suction versus abdominoplasty. Aesthetic Plast Surg 9:265, 1985.

Baran NK, Celebi C. A ten year experience with reduction mammaplasty and abdominoplasty. What is happening in our part of the world? Clin Plast Surg 11:479, 1984.

Barett BM, Kelly MV. Combined abdominoplasty and augmentation mammaplasty through a transverse suprapubic incision. Ann Plast Surg 4:286, 1980.

Baroudi R, Kepke EM, Carvalho CG. Abdominoplasty. Plast Reconstr Surg 54:161, 1974.

Baroudi R, Kepke EM, Carvalho CG. Mammary reduction combined with reverse abdominoplasty. Ann Plast Surg 2:368, 1979.

Barraya L, Napkane E. Abdomen molluscum. Abdomen pendulum. Reparation. Nouvel ombilic. Presse Med 48:2287, 1968.

Biesenberger H. Abdomen pendulous. Zentralbl Chir 63:1399, 1936.

Bozola AR, Psillakis JM. Abdominoplasty: A new concept and classification for treatment. Plast Reconstr Surg 82:983, 1988.

Boyd J, Taylor G, Corleti R. The vascular territories of the superior and the deep inferior epigastric systems. Plast Reconstr Surg 73:1, 1984.

Callia W. Contribuicao para o estudo da correcao em cirurgica do abdomen pendulo e globoso tecnica original. These Med, Sao Paulo, 1965.

Callia WEP. Uma plastica para o cirurgiao geral. Med Hosp 1:40, 1967.

Caravel JB. Plasties abdominales. Technique personelle de reconstruction ombilicale. Report de la cicatrice au fond de l'omlilic. Ann Chir Plast Esthet 26:289, 1981.

Cardoso de Castro C, Daher M. Simultaneous reduction mammaplasty and abdominoplasty. Plast Reconstr Surg 61:36, 1978.

Cardoso de Castro C, Cupello AMB, Cintra H. Limited incisions in abdominoplasty. Ann Plast Surg 19:436, 1987.

Christman KD. Death following suction lipectomy and abdominoplasty. Plast Reconstr Surg 78:428, 1986.

Correa Iturraspe M. Dermolipectomia vertical del abdomen. Bol Soc Argent Cirj 13:648, 1952.

Davis TW. Morbid obesity. Clin Plast Surg 11:517, 1984.

De la Plaza R, Arrojo JM. The rationalization of liposuction. Toward a safer and more accurate technique. Aesthetic Plast Surg 13:243, 1989.

Delfino M, Appiani, E. Association of Psillakis-Appiani technique. Personal communication, Argentina, 1989.

Dellon AL. Fleur de lis abdominoplasty. Aesthetic Plast Surg 9:27, 1985.

Depaulis J. La chirurgie des abdomens pendulums. Reflexions sur 20 cas. J Med Bordeaux 144:697, 1967.

Donnabella P. Defatting in the epigastric region. Personal communication, 1980.

Dubou R, Ousterhout DK. Placement of the umbilicus in an abdominoplasty. Plast Reconstr Surg 61:291, 1978.

Elbaz JS. A propos des plasties abdominales. Technique de "fer a cheval." Ann Chir Plast 19:155, 1974.

Elbaz JS, Flageul G. Plastic surgery of the abdomen. New York: Masson USA, 1978.

Elbaz JS, Flageul G. Liposuction et chirurgie plastique de l'abdomen. Paris: Masson, 1989.

Enderby GEH. Hypotensive anesthesia in surgery. Ann R Coll Surg Engl 11:11 1952.

Enderby GEH. The advantages of controlled hypotension in surgery. Br Med Bull 14:1 1958.

Elsahy N. Abdominoplasty combined with correction of the flaccidity of the lateral lower abdomen and the flanks. Aesthetic Plast Surg 9:33, 1985.

Fischi RA. Vertical abdominoplasty. Plast Reconstr Surg 51:139, 1973.

Franco T, Associacao de abdominoplastia e cirurgia intra-cavitaria. Rev Bras Cir 6:15, 1978.

Freeman BS, Weimer DR. Abdominoplasty with special attention to the construction of the umbilicus. Technique and complications. Aesthetic Plast Surg 2:65, 1978.

Goldwyn R. Abdominoplasty as a combined procedure: Added benefit or double trouble? Plast Reconstr Surg, 78:383, 1986.

Gonzales Ulloa M. Belt lipectomy. Br J Plast Surg 13:179, 1960.

Grazer FM, Goldwyn RM. Abdominoplasty assessed by survey with emphasis on complications. Plast Reconstr Surg 59:513, 1977.

Grazer FM. Suction-assisted lipectomy, suction lipectomy, lipolysis and lipexeresis. Plast Reconstr Surg 72:620, 1983.

Greminger RF. The Mini-abdominoplasty. Plast Reconstr Surg 79:356, 1987.

Guerrerosantos J, Dicksheet S, Carillo C, Sandoval M. Umbilical reconstruction with secondary abdominoplasty. Ann Plast Surg 5:139, 1980.

Hakme F. Abdominoplasty: Peri and supraumbilical lipectomy. Aesthetic Plast Surg 7:213, 1983.

Hodgkinson DJ. Umbilicoplasty: Conversion of "outie" to "innie." Aesthetic Plast Surg 7:221, 1983.

Illouz YG. Body contouring by lipolysis: A 5-year experience with over 3000 cases. Plast Reconstr Surg 72:591, 1983.

Isaacs G. Breast shaping procedures, abdominoplasty and thighplasty in Australia. Clin Plast Surg 11:525, 1984.

Jackson IT, Downie PA. Abdominoplasty: The waistline stitch and other refinements. Plast Reconstr Surg 61:180, 1978.

Jamra FA. Reconstruction of the umbilicus by a double VY procedure. Plast Reconstr Surg 64:106, 1979.

Juri J, Juri C, Raiden G. Reconstruction of the umbilicus in abdominoplasty. Plast Reconstr Surg 63:580, 1979.

Kamper MJ, Dwight V, Galooway DV, Aschley F. Abdominal panniculectomy after massive weight loss. Plast Reconstr Surg 50:441, 1972.

Kesselring UK, Meyer R. Suction curette for removal of excessive local deposits of subcutaneous fat. Plast Reconstr Surg 62:305, 1978.

Lewis CM. Early experience of aspirative lipoplasty of the abdomen. Aesthetic Plast Surg 11:33, 1987.

McIndoe A. Hypotensive anaesthesia in surgery. Plast Reconstr Surg 17:332, 1956.

Patel HP. Hypotensive Anaesthesia. Bailliere's Clin Anaesthesiol 1:9, 1987.

Pitanguy I. Abdominal lipectomy: An approach to it through an analysis of 300 consecutive cases. Plast Reconstr Surg 40:384, 1967.

Planas J. The "vest over pants" abdominoplasty. Plast Reconstr Surg 61:694, 1978.

Pompeo de Pina D. Aesthetic abdominal deformities: A personal approach to the posterior rectus sheath and rectus muscles. Plast Reconstr Surg 75:660, 1985.

Pontes R. Defatting of the flap in abdominoplasty in obese patients. Personal communication, 1981.

Psillakis JM. Abdominoplasty: Some ideas to improve results. Aesthetic Plast Surg 2:205, 1978.

Psillakis JM. Plastic surgery of the abdomen with improvement in the body contour. Clin Plast Surg 11:3, 1984.

Psillakis JM. Abdominoplasty: Treatment of the external oblique muscle to obtain a better waist. Ann J SulBras Plast Surg S.B.C.P., 1984, p 85.

Psillakis JM. Abdominoplasty: Classification and concepts. Plastic Surgery Educational Foundation. Advanced Body Contouring Symposium, Newport Beach, California, 1987.

Psillakis JM. Abdominoplasty: A new classification and the "lyre form" of the abdomen. Manhattan Eye, Ear, Nose and Throat Hospital Symposium, Institute of Reconstructive Surgery, New York, 1988.

Rebello C, Franco T. Abdominoplasty through a submammary incision. Rev Bras Cir 62:249, 1972.

Regnault P. Abdominoplasty by the W technique. Plast Reconstr Surg 55:272, 1975.

Robertson JI. Complication of "dermolipectomy" as an encore to abdominal operative procedure. S Afr Med J 56:141, 1979.

Schepelmann E. Ueber Baucheenkenplastik mit Besonderer. Beruksichtigung des Hangebauches. Beitr Klin Chir 111:272, 1918.

Schrude J. Lipexeresis or a means of eliminating local adiposity. Aesthetic Plast Surg 4:215, 1980.

Schurte M, Letterman G. Abdominoplasty or abdominal dermolipectomy. Ann Plast Surg 2:235, 1979.

Serson ND. Abdominoplasty. Aesthetic Plast Surg 6:1, 1982.

Souza Pinto EF. A new methodology in abdominal aesthetic surgery. Aesthetic Plast Surg 11:213, 1987.

Stuckey JG. Midabdomen abdominoplasty. Plast Reconstr Surg 63:333, 1979.

Thorek M. Plastic surgery of the breast and abdominal wall. Springfield, IL: Charles C Thomas, 1942, p 11.

Vilain R, Dubousset J. Technique et indications de la lipectomie circulaire. Ann Chir 18:289, 1964.

Vilain R, Dardour JC, Staub S, Mitz V. Dix questions a propos de l'aspiration de la graisse par la technique d'Y.G. Illouz. Ann Chir Plast Esthet 29:180, 1984.

Wilkinson TS, Schwartz BE. Individual modifications in body contour surgery: The "limited" abdominoplasty. Plast Reconstr Surg 77:779, 1986.

Index